A Colour Atlas of
Injury in Sport

J. G. P. Williams
MA, MSc, MB, BChir, FRCS, DPhysMed

Medical Director,
Farnham Park Rehabilitation Centre
Consultant in Rehabilitation Medicine,
Wexham Park Hospital, Slough
Formerly Honorary Secretary,
British Association of Sport and Medicine
Secretary General, International Federation
of Sports Medicine

Wolfe Medical Publications Ltd

Copyright © John G. P. Williams, 1980
Published by Wolfe Medical Publications Ltd, 1980
Printed by Smeets-Weert, Holland
ISBN 0 7234 0736 3

This book is one of the titles in the series of
Wolfe Medical Atlases, a series which brings
together probably the world's largest systematic
published collection of diagnostic colour
photographs.
For a full list of Atlases in the series, plus
forthcoming titles and details of our surgical,
dental and veterinary Atlases, please write to
Wolfe Medical Publications Ltd, Wolfe House,
3 Conway Street, London W1P 6HE.

General Editor, Wolfe Medical Atlases:
G. Barry Carruthers, MD(Lond)

Contents

(continued)

Introduction

The material in this atlas forms the basis of lectures on injury in sport presented at instruction courses in the United Kingdom and abroad. Attention is focused primarily on those injuries which are peculiar to sport and seldom encountered outside the sporting context. However, injuries of wider incidence are also included, though in less detail, where they have a particular relevance to sport, for example, severe ligament injuries of the knee joint.

Inevitably in a small atlas it is not possible to be exhaustive, but the more common problems are all included, with a selection of those rarities which makes the care of injured sportsmen so fascinating. Where the conditions concerned are not amenable to clinical photography, for example the anterior tibial compartment syndrome, the salient features are illustrated by diagram, and in many instances are further illustrated by radiographical, operative, or histological material. Nearly all the clinical conditions presented have been observed in the Regional Centre for Sports Injuries of the Oxford Regional Health Authority based on Farnham Park Rehabilitation Centre but inevitably it has not proved possible to provide from local resources suitable photographs in every instance. I have been very fortunate in obtaining excellent additional illustrations the better to exemplify many of the conditions, and for their help and cooperation I am deeply grateful to those friends and colleagues whose names are listed in the acknowledgements.

Considerations of space demand that comments on treatment are restricted to the less common conditions, and those where there are particularly useful alterations to established lines. Methods of treatment for most of these injuries are well defined and details readily available from other sources. The primary consideration in management is essentially restoration of maximum function in minimum time.

I hope this little atlas will serve to demonstrate the extraordinarily wide range of clinical problems associated with sport, many of which do form an important part of everyday accident or orthopaedic practice.

Acknowledgements

I would like to thank my friends and colleagues:

Barbara Ansell, David Bell, Sue Boardman, John Buck, Graeme Campbell, Sheila Christian, John Davies, Patrick England, Ennis Giordani, David Hirschowitz, Jack Kanski, Philip Kerr, Chris Lewis, James Moncur, Robert Nagle, Nigel Tubbs and Leon Walkden for additional material,

Andrew Dent for helping to put it all together,

The Editors of *Sports Medicine, Medisport, British Journal of Sports Medicine, Journal of Bone and Joint Surgery* and *Medicine* for permission to use material previously published;

Derek Griffin, Clinical Photographer at Wexham Park Hospital, for his help with the clinical photographs, and

Don Morley and Tony Duffy of All Sport for their magnificent portfolio of colour action photographs which give real life to the Atlas.

for Sally,
Stephen, Philippa and David,
with love

1 Nature and incidence of injury in sport

The term 'sports injury' is something of a misnomer. Injury is the result of the application to the body or part of the body of forces which exceed the body's ability to adjust to them. These forces may be applied instantaneously or over a considerable period. The exact nature of the injury (1) – the tissues involved and the way in which the damage is sustained – depends upon the mechanism by which excess force is applied. The body is able to differentiate between different types of stress (for example the tissue response to a direct blow is different from that to a sudden stretch), but it is not able to differentiate between the different activities in which one particular mechanical type of violence is applied.

Most injuries sustained in sport are essentially no different from those sustained in other activities, although the demands of the patient in terms of rehabilitation and return to activity may be significantly greater.

From a practical point of view studies of patients attending clinics for sports injuries (2) show that a very substantial majority of problems could be well handled either by general practitioners, hospital accident and emergency departments, or hospital specialists in appropriate disciplines as part of their normal practice.

The number of injuries and clinical problems which are peculiar to sport as such and which are in general unrelated to ordinary day-to-day activities is small, but they do require particular expertise and knowledge in their management.

1   The causal chain in injury.

2

A. Patients suitable for treatment by General Practitioner or Casualty Officer	± 65%
B. Patients requiring orthodox specialist attention, e.g. orthopaedic, rheumatological, etc.	± 25%
C. Patients requiring **specialised sports** medical attention	± 10%
	100%

2   **Clinical management categories** of cases presenting with sports injuries.

Classification of injury by causal factors

Consequential   (due to sports participation)

  Primary   (direct result of sporting stress)

    Extrinsic   (due to external violence)

      Human   (e.g. body-contact sports)

      Implemental   (e.g. racquet sports, gymnastics)

        Instantaneous   (due to immediate violence)

        Overuse   (due to repeated stress)

      Vehicular   (e.g. motor car accident)

      Environmental   (e.g. mountaineering accident, water sport accident)

    Intrinsic   (due to stress developed *within* victim)

      Instantaneous

      Overuse

      Acute   (occurring in one incident of overuse)

      Chronic   (developing over a long period)

  Secondary   (as a result of an earlier, often inadequately treated injury in sport)

    Early   (developing soon after primary injury)

    Late   (developing many years after injury)

Non consequential   (injuries and other conditions not directly caused by sporting stress, but which are influenced by it and interfere with sports participation)

The extent and severity of the injury is modified by a number of factors including the general physical and psychological fitness of the patient, his constitutional suitability for the sport, environmental conditions at the time of the injury, age and sex and general level of nutrition. The victim's general level of skill and proficiency is also significant. It is interesting to note how in body-contact sport most severe injuries occur in the first quarter of the game, whereas the last quarter of the game is marked by an excessive number of minor and relatively trivial injuries exacerbated by the players' fatigue.

How different types of injury happen

3

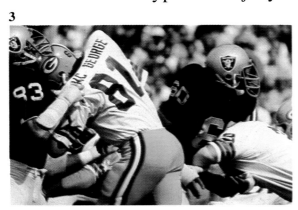

4

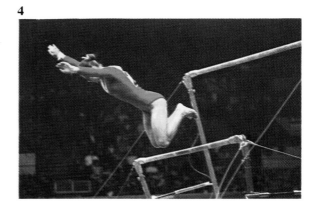

3 Tackle in American football. Direct body contact violence (extrinsic – human).

4 Asymmetric bars collapse as Tourischeva dismounts. Nearly a nasty accident (extrinsic – implemental).

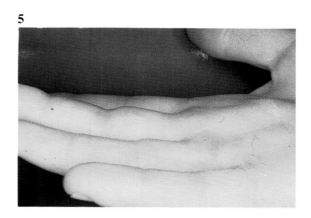

5 **Callosity** overlying trigger finger in fencer (extrinsic implemental overuse injury).

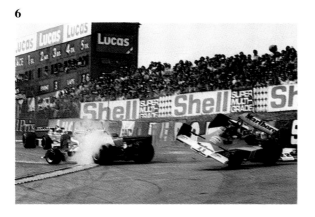

6 **Crash in motor race** (extrinsic vehicular).

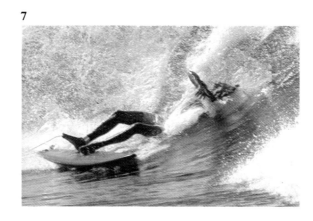

7 **Surfer 'wipes out'** (extrinsic environmental).

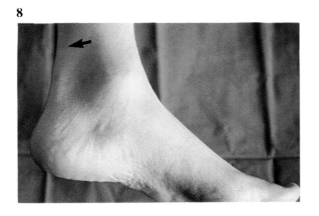

8 **Complete rupture of tendo Achilles** in runner (instantaneous intrinsic injury). Note 'dent' in tendon above distal stump.

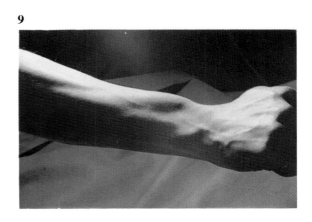

9 **Tenosynovitis.** Four days after winning the 129-mile Devizes to Westminster cause race. Tenosynovitis of the forearm extensor (acute intrinsic overuse injury).

11

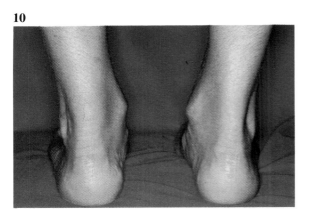

10 Achilles tendonitis in long-distance runner (chronic intrinsic overuse injury).

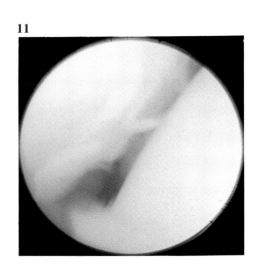

11 Chondromalacia patellae (arthroscopic appearance) (early secondary condition).

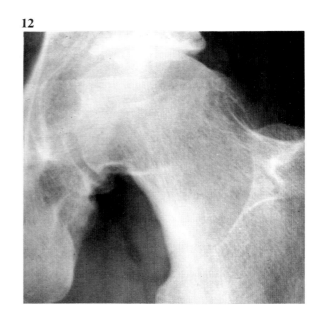

12 Osteoarthrosis of the hip in a race walker (late secondary condition).

Generally, as would be expected, extrinsic injuries produce more severe tissue damage than intrinsic because the forces involved are substantially greater. In intrinsic injury the key causes are either breakdown of technique under stress (which leads to instantaneous injury) or the overlong or too great application of training or competition stresses (which produces overuse injury). In the management of intrinsic injury, therefore, correction of any technical faults in the practice of the sport, with modification of the training programme, is an essential component of patient management.

2 Types of tissue damage

Tissue response to injury largely reflects the nature of the damaging mechanism. The pattern of injury throughout the various tissues involved will tend to a degree of uniformity with some variation at individual sites as a response to peculiar local factors. The general pattern of injury, however, remains reasonably constant throughout the body. Typical examples of pathological response to trauma in the tissues are repeatedly reproduced at different anatomical sites.

Skin injury

A variety of different types of trauma may be noted.

A laceration is damage to the skin involving the full thickness and exposing the underlying subcutaneous tissue.

An abrasion or graze is an injury, often of the glancing type, where the surface of the skin is broken but there is no complete tear throughout the whole depth.

A haematoma, contusion or bruise is due to a direct blow on the surface, usually with a blunt instrument.

Puncture wounds are lacerations where the depth of the wound is greater than its length or breadth. They are typically the result of injury with a pointed instrument.

Burns involve damage to the skin as a result of heat. In friction burns invariably an abrasive component is present as well.

Blisters are injuries to the skin where one layer is detached from the layer beneath, the gap between becoming filled with a serious fluid exuded by the injured cells.

Blistering does not occur if the load is built up gradually, allowing the skin to adapt.

Skin damage may show a mixture of injury, for example bruising and laceration together.

13

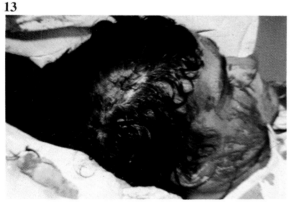

13 Scalp laceration through full thickness of skin. Implement was the studs of a rugby boot.

14

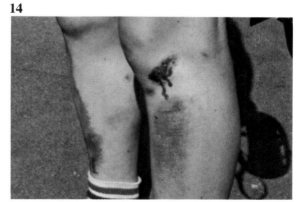

14 Abrasion due to direct violence – leg injuries to a cyclist after a fall in a road race.

15

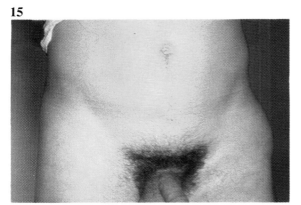

15 Haematoma. Bruising over the left iliac crest in a footballer after a collision on the field.

16

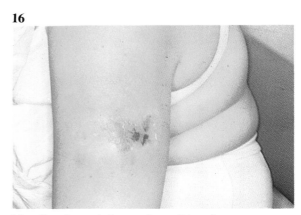

16 Crush and laceration. Bite from an angry horse.

17

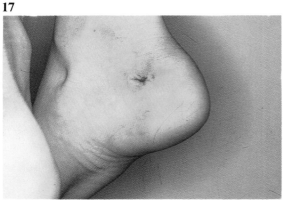

17 Puncture wound. Injury to the heel as a result of dog bite in a runner waylaid by an irascible dog while out training! If a dog shows signs of aggression walk slowly. Don't run!

18

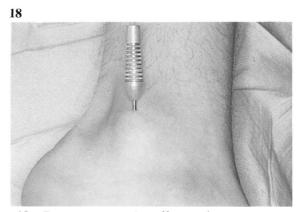

18 Puncture wound – off target!

19

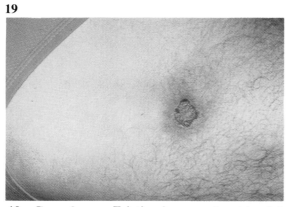

19 Grass burns. Friction burn on the skin of the thigh over the greater trochanter, caused by a sliding fall on hard ground. These burns commonly become secondarily infected.

20

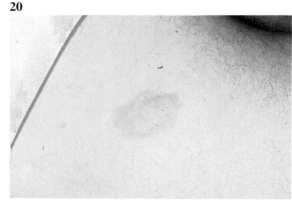

20 Hypertrophic scarring over the greater trochanter in a friction burn (in this case a cyclist fell during a track race) that healed with excessive scar-tissue formation.

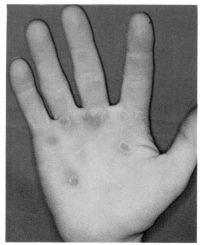

21 **Blistered hands.** As in other tissues the response to overuse is injury – blisters on the palms of an oarsman resuming training after a break.

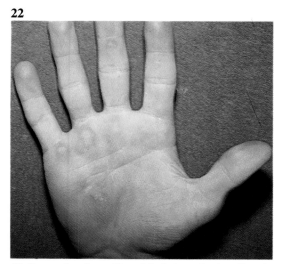

22 **Calloused palms.** Provided that the loading is built up gradually and progressively, tissues can adapt to high levels of use – callosities on the hands of an international gymnast.

Muscle injury/muscle tear: types

Muscle damage occurs as a result of either external forces (contusion, haematoma or laceration) or more commonly as the result of forces generated within the tissue, i.e. as an intrinsic injury. The injury is then called a strain or tear of which there are three basic types, complete and partial, the latter being either interstitial or intramuscular.

The severity of muscle injury will depend very often on the degree of training of the individual. The fully fit athlete who is properly stretched before competing and who has an adequate technique will seldom get injured. In the fit subject bleeding is more marked but resolution subsequently more rapid. A history of chronic muscle tear invariably delays resumption of sport.

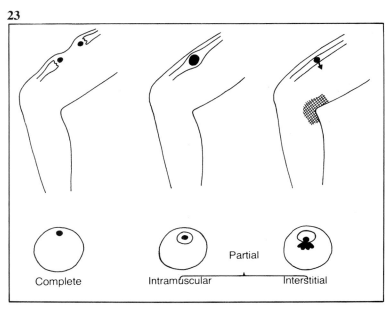

23 **Differential classification** of muscle tear.

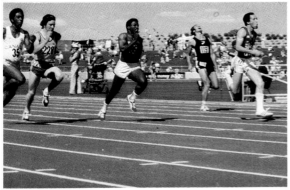

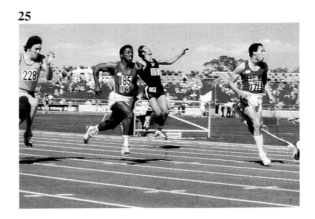

24 and 25 Action sequence – a muscle tear as it happens. Note runner in black strip.

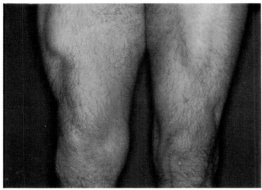

26 Example of complete muscle rupture in a rugby player (rectus femoris).

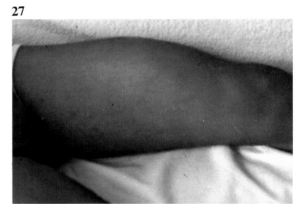

27 Example of intramuscular injury showing marked swelling of the muscle – footballer (quadriceps).

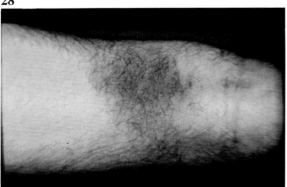

28 Example of interstitial injury showing extravasation of blood – sprinter (hamstring).

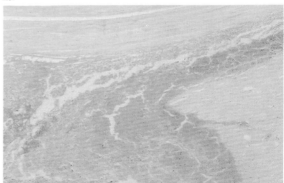

29 Muscle haematoma – histology.

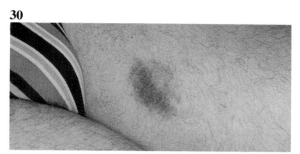

30 Muscle haematoma. Extrinsic injury – blow from a hockey ball.

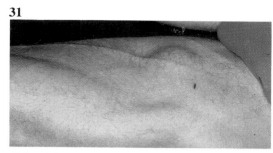

31 Muscle hernia. Muscle tissue bulging up under pressure through split in overlying fascia (abductor). Probably an old interstitial tear.

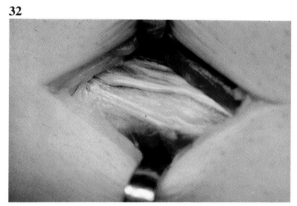

32 Muscle shortening. Typically due to contraction of excess scar tissue in an inadequately treated partial tear (appearance at operation) (gastrocnemius).

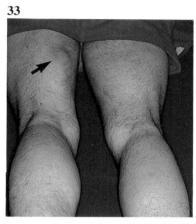

33 Muscle spasm (associated with joint injury). Note apparent tightness in the hamstrings. This patient had sustained a knee injury with inability to extend the knee fully – this is not due to locking but rather due to muscle spasm. Not to be confused with muscle shortening associated with muscle injury.

34 Loss of extensibility. Patient with recent injury of the right quadriceps showing (**a**) normal side with knee fully flexed and hip fully extended and (**b**) abnormal side – the hip is not fully extended and the knee is not fully flexed.

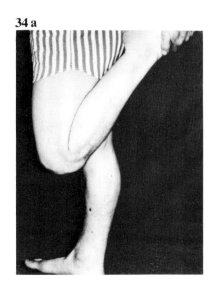

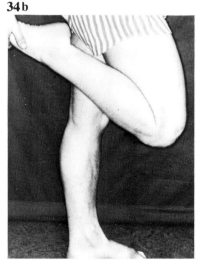

Ectopic calcification

Otherwise known as myositis ossificans, this is a condition in which deposits of calcium and eventually bone are laid down in the muscle, usually as a result of a direct *blow*. Does not occur as a rule with intrinsic injury. May be induced by over-vigorous treatment (especially massage and passive stretching) of a muscle haematoma.

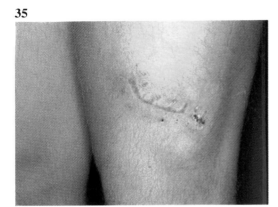

35 **Haematoma.** Thigh of a cyclist who fell from his bicycle and sustained a massive haematoma of the front of the thigh and a laceration. The haematoma subsequently developed ectopic calcification.

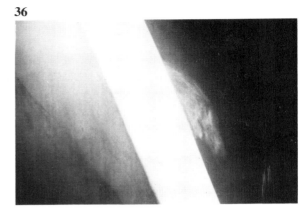

36 **Radiograph showing ectopic calcification** in the front of the thigh.

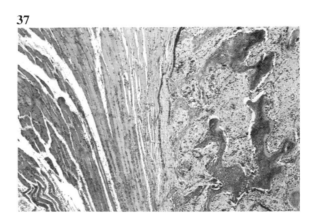

37 **Ectopic calcification or myositis ossificans.** Histological appearance.

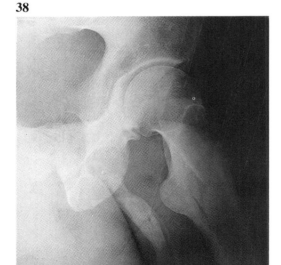

38 **Ectopic calcification.** Radiograph showing well-defined bone formation in the adductor of a rugby player.

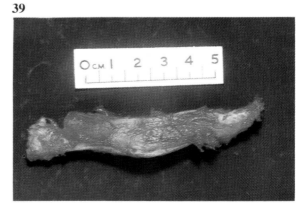

39 **Ectopic bone.** Operation specimen. After removal of the ectopic bone, the individual was able to resume rugby football.

Myositis ossificans

40 to 45 Myositis ossificans affecting the quadriceps on the front of the thigh – serial xrays showing development and resolution of ectopic calcification in a young footballer after a blow on the front of the thigh.

Note time span for resolution.

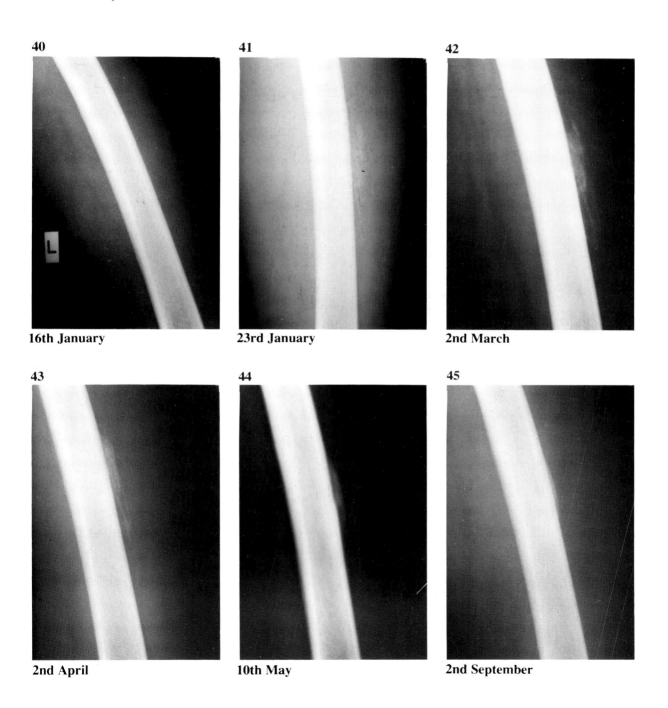

40

16th January

41

23rd January

42

2nd March

43

2nd April

44

10th May

45

2nd September

Tendon injury

In sport damage to tendons by direct violence is uncommon. Usually injuries are intrinsic and most are of the overuse type. They are readily classified by their local pathology which is associated with well-defined clinical features.

Diagnosis	Key features
Rupture – complete	Sudden onset Gap in tendon
Rupture – partial	Sudden onset No gap in tendon
Focal degeneration	Gradual onset Well localised tenderness Minimal swelling Moves with tendon
Tendonitis	Gradual onset Diffuse tenderness Well-marked swelling Moves with tendon
Peritendonitis – acute	Rapid onset Crepitus Diffuse swelling Does not move with tendon
Peritendonitis – chronic	Slow onset – often with repeated episodes Localised thickening Does not move with tendon
Mixed lesion	Mixed features

46 Types of lesion. Classification of types of tendon lesion and key clinical features.

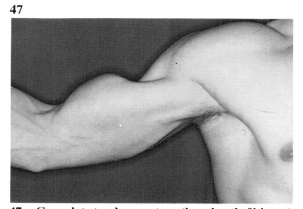

47 Complete tendon rupture (long head of biceps). Tendon ends are separated by the pull of the attached muscle which becomes virtually non-functional.

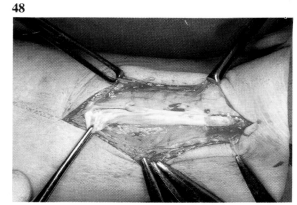

48 Partial tendon rupture (Achilles tendon). Muscle function not mechanically impaired as a rule but inhibited by pain.

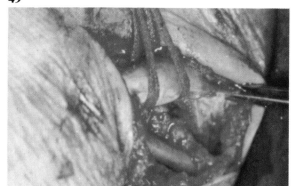

49   **Focal degeneration with calcification (tibialis posterior tendon).** Clinically and functionally similar to partial rupture of which it is the overuse variant.

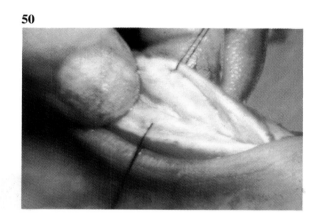

50   **Tendonitis (Achilles tendon).** Generalised oedema and inflammation of the tendon causing variable pain and loss of function.

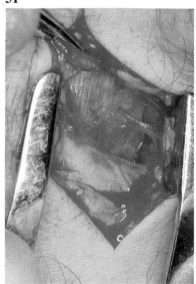

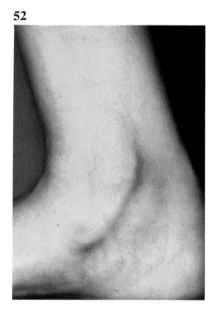

51   **Peritendonitis (patellar tendon).** May be acute or chronic and is an overuse injury characterised by initially oedema and later fibrosis in tissues surrounding the tendon. Adhesion to surrounding structures is common.

52   **Tendovaginitis (tibialis posterior).** Usually a chronic inflammation with fibrosis and stenosis of the tendon sheath.

Joint injury

Joint injuries are common in sport, particularly in body-contact events. The range of damage varies from minor sprain to major fracture or dislocation. Most joints are synovial, being reinforced in certain sites by ligaments, and some contain fibro-cartilaginous menisci. Damage may occur to any or all of these structures. Traumatic synovitis occurs as the result of joint injury in which the lining membrane or synovium is damaged. Where the damage is severe the response is acute and haemorrhagic, where damage is less severe the response is a serous effusion.

Traumatic synovitis

53

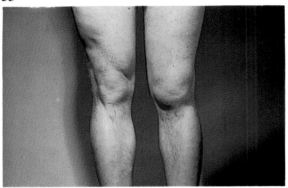

53 Clinical appearance showing swelling and effusion in the left knee, after a rugby injury.

54

	Synovial effusion	Haemarthrosis
Onset	Delayed ± 12hrs	Immediate
Tension	Usually slight	Considerable
Volume	Usually small (50ml −)	Large (50ml +)
Severity of injury	+ → ++	++ → +++ ++

54 Differential diagnosis in joint effusion.

55

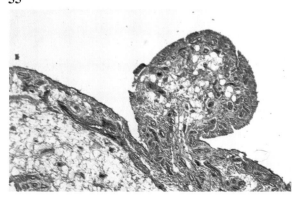

55 Histology of villus in low grade traumatic synovitis.

56

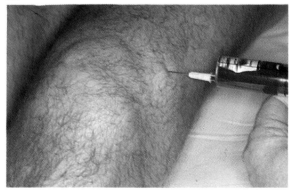

56 Haemarthrosis – aspiration of blood-stained synovial fluid from the knee of a footballer.

Loose bodies

Loose bodies are a common cause of joint problems in sport, usually because they interfere mechanically with the function of the joint. In some instances, as in osteochondritis dissecans, discomfort in the joint may be associated with the underlying condition.

57

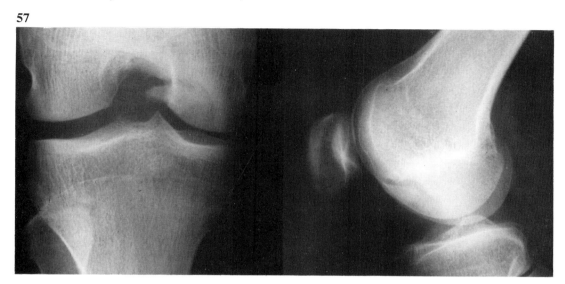

57 Osteochondritis dissecans. Loose body is commonly the result of earlier osteochrondritis dissecans; in this case the medial femoral condyle is involved.

58

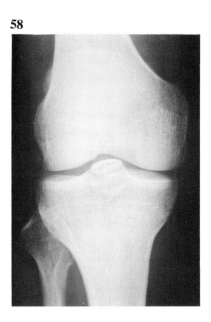

58 Radiograph of loose body. In this instance caused by an old fracture of the anterior tibial spine.

59

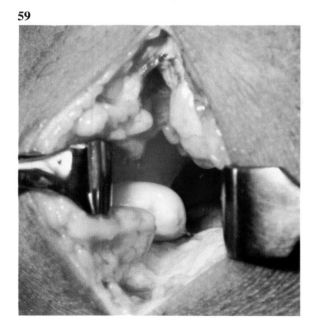

59 Loose body demonstrated at operation – removed because it was causing locking.

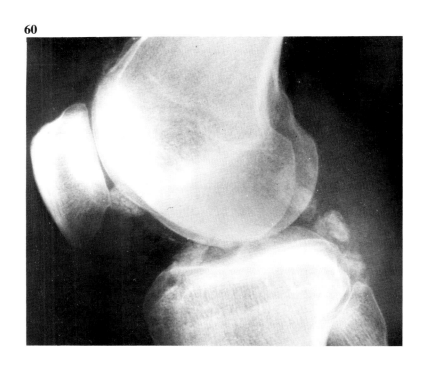

60 Osteochondromatosis. Multiple loose bodies.

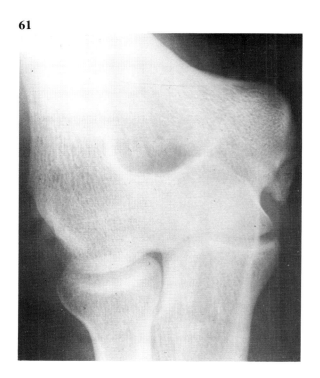

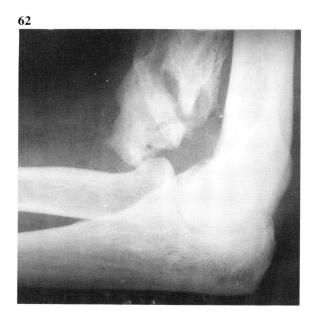

61 Golfer's elbow. Capsular calcification (golfer's elbow), which must not be confused with intra-capsular loose body.

62 Ectopic calcification, abnormal bone deposits on the anterior aspect of the elbow joint, superficial but attached to the capsule.

Ligament injury

Damage to ligaments may cause minor tears, stretching or complete rupture. Complete rupture leads to mechanical instability. Tearing, even if quite minor, may damage the proprioceptive feedback mechanism and lead to stable instability.

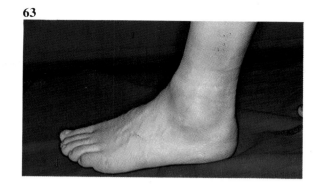
63

63 Sprain. A traction injury to a ligament without loss of continuity.

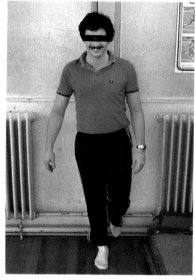
64 a

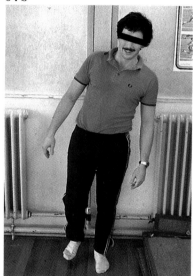
64 b

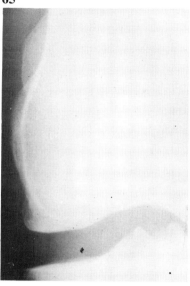
65

64a and b Stable instability. Loss of proprioception in left ankle joint (normal side (**a**) for comparison) as a result of ligament injury with no gross mechanical instability. Note inability of patient to balance properly on affected ankle.

65 Ligament rupture with loss of continuity and mechanical instability.

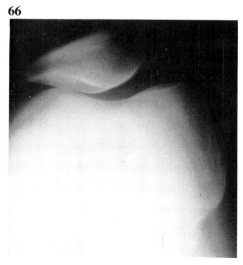
66

66 Subluxation. Misalignment of joint surface but some overlap.

Dislocation is often associated with severe ligamentous injury leading to instability. In some cases, particularly around the elbow joint, damage leads during the recovery phase to ectopic calcification and subsequent limitation in joint function.

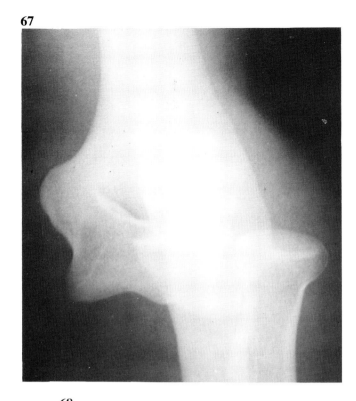

67 Dislocation. Complete disruption of joint surface contact.

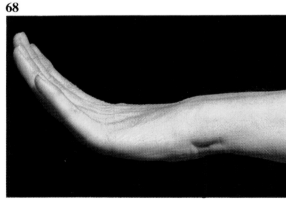

68 Hypermobility. Excessive laxity or 'double jointedness' may be so severe as to be pathological, and is a contraindication to body-contact sports and those requiring excess mobility (e.g. gymnastics and trampolining), especially in children.

Other soft tissue injury of any severity is happily quite rare in sport and usually the result of direct violence.

Vascular injury

Vascular injury usually complicates other injury but is occasionally isolated. These conditions usually occur as result of direct blow or wound. Spontaneous arterial thrombosis has been described but is probably due to intimal damage. Later aneurysm or arteriovenous fistula may form.

Venous thrombosis is much more common, often associated with an episode of overuse. No specific sites are particularly implicated but the lower limb is more usually involved. Congenital anomalies (e.g. compression due to cervical rib) may present in or effects be exacerbated by sport.

Nerve injury

The commonest type of nerve injury is neuropraxia caused by a direct blow, e.g. over ulnar nerve at elbow or lateral popliteal nerve at fibula neck. More severe damage may complicate lacerations (division of nerve) and fractures and dislocations. Overuse injury is rare but includes ulnar neuritis in throwers. The most usual sites are illustrated below.

69

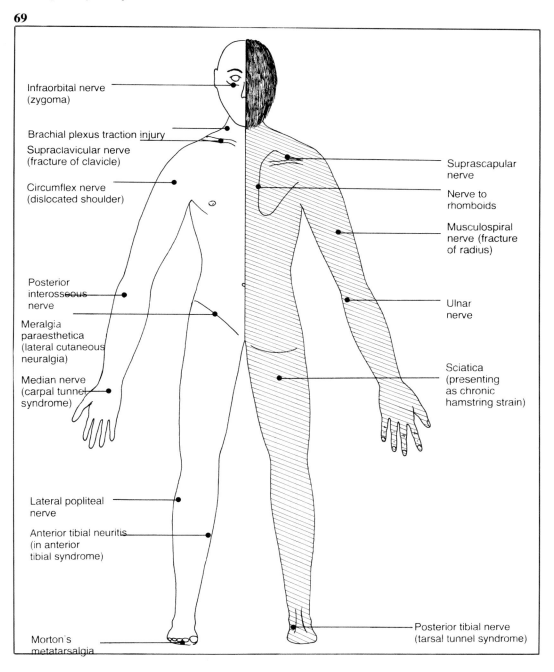

Infraorbital nerve
(zygoma)

Brachial plexus traction injury

Supraclavicular nerve
(fracture of clavicle)

Circumflex nerve
(dislocated shoulder)

Posterior
interosseous
nerve

Meralgia
paraesthetica
(lateral cutaneous
neuralgia)

Median nerve
(carpal tunnel
syndrome)

Lateral popliteal
nerve

Anterior tibial neuritis
(in anterior
tibial syndrome)

Morton's
metatarsalgia

Suprascapular
nerve

Nerve to
rhomboids

Musculospiral
nerve (fracture
of radius)

Ulnar
nerve

Sciatica
(presenting
as chronic
hamstring strain)

Posterior tibial nerve
(tarsal tunnel syndrome)

69   Common sites of nerve injury caused in sport.

Bone injury

Bone injuries are quite common in sport, usually as a result of direct violence (sometimes deliberate!). Generally fractures sustained in sport differ little from those sustained in other activities. Treatment may have to be more vigorous, particularly during the rehabilitation phase, and in some instances internal fixation (e.g. with compression plating) may be the treatment of choice to diminish the disability period.

Instantaneous fracture

70a

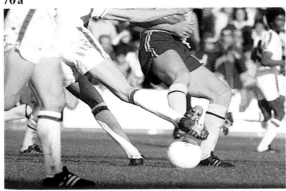

70b

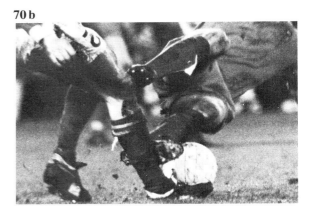

70a and b How it happens (**a**) A player 'going over the top'. This may occur accidentally but (**b**) too often is a deliberate foul.

71

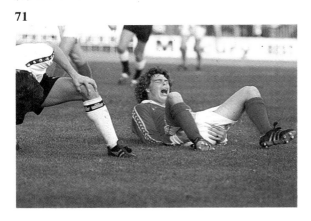

71 A football player breaks his leg.

72

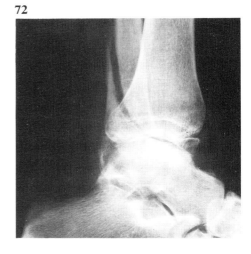

72 Fractured fibula. A football accident. Note also impingement exostosis on anterior tibial joint margin (see **445**).

Subchondral fracture

Occasionally there may be bony damage beneath the articular cartilage (a common site is the knee) associated with ligament injury or with the presence of a loose body jamming between the joint surfaces. Diagnosis is often problematical as the defect may be extremely difficult to pick up radiologically.

Stress fracture

Stress fractures of the tibia, fibula and metatarsals are very common in sport as a result of excessive training on hard surfaces.

73

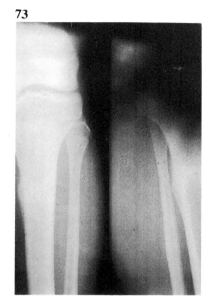

74

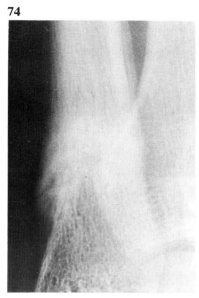

75

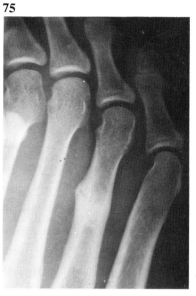

73 Stress fracture of tibia.

74 Stress fracture of fibula.

75 Stress fracture of metatarsal ('march' fracture).

Pathological fracture

77

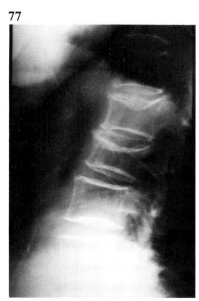

76

76 Osteochondritis or epiphysitis is more common in children. Sever's disease of the calcaneal apophysis is an overuse injury caused by excessive training in the adolescent patient.

77 Wedge fracture in osteoporosis. This elderly patient tripped on a bowling green.

3 Other conditions presenting as sports injuries

THE POSSIBILITY THAT AN APPARENT INJURY IN SPORT MAY BE THE FIRST SIGN OF SOME SINISTER CONDITION SHOULD ALWAYS BE REMEMBERED.

Infection

Infections may appear as sports injuries. The patient presents having first experienced pain in the affected tissue during sporting activity (when local blood supply is greater than at rest).

78 Septic arthritis. Radiograph of the wrist of an international athlete with a septic arthritis. After treatment he was able to return to international competition. Note severe decalcification.

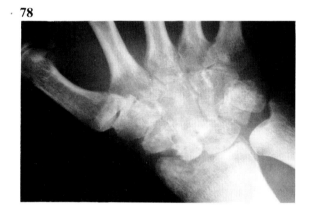
78

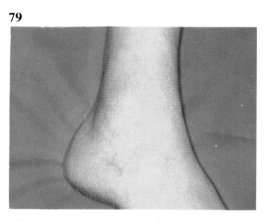
79

79 Acute osteomyelitis in the lower end of the fibula in a young rugby player. Initial presentation suggested a stress fracture – note swelling over lateral malleolus.

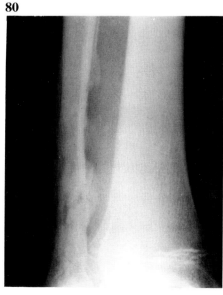
80

80 Radiological appearance (of **79**) one month after onset. The patient has now returned to active sport with no disability.

Tumours

Tumours may present as sports injuries.

Benign tumours

81

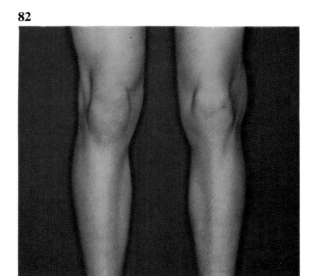

81 Solitary exostosis on lower end of femur
interfering with vastus medialis function in a young
swimmer.

82

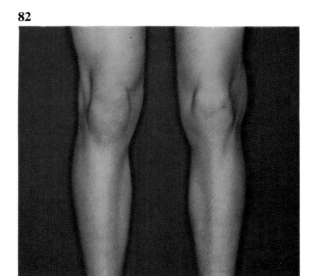

82 Cavernous haemangioma on the outer side of
the left knee in a teenage track athlete. This was an
extensive lesion spreading down into the popliteal
fossa and through the lateral head of gastrocnemius.

Borderline

83

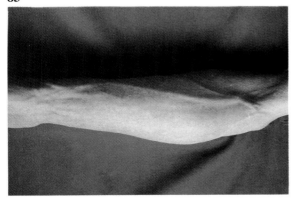

84

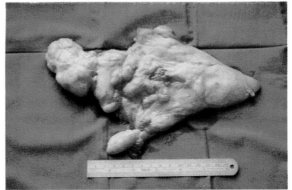

83 and 84 Lipoma with some primitive cells
previously diagnosed as a 'muscle tear' in an angler.

Malignant tumours

Malignant connective tissue tumours are uncommon but prognosis tends to be bad so that early detection is essential to reduce mortality rate. The possibility that a malignant tumour may present as a sports injury should always be remembered. A high index of suspicion will lead to early diagnosis and perhaps avoidance of tragedy.

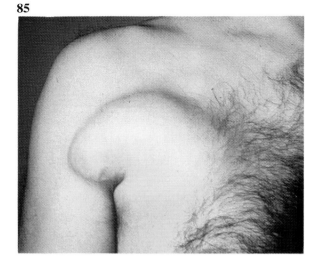
85

85   Rhabdomyosarcoma of the pectoralis major.

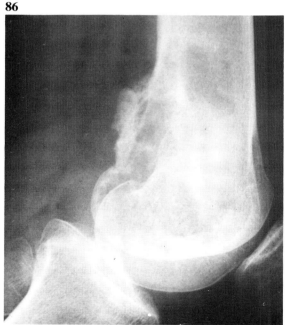
86

86   Giant cell tumour – radiograph of lower end of femur.

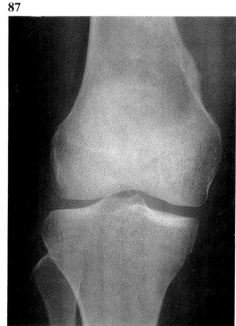
87

87   Radiograph showing osteosarcoma in the femur of a schoolgirl, presenting as pain in the knee after netball.

4 Head and facial injuries

Head injury

Head injuries are too common. They involve transient dazing, or periods of unconsciousness with more or less severe brain damage. They occur in body-contact and vehicular sports and in hardball games. Adequate headgear may not fully protect. Emergency resuscitation may be needed.

88 Transient dazing is common. Patient usually responds well to a cold douche.

88

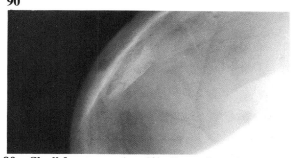

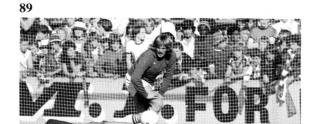

89 Concussion may occur when there are heavy impacts in body-contact sport, e.g. in a clash of heads.

90 Skull fracture. A golf ball may be a dangerous missile. Depressed fracture of the skull; radiograph of a victim of a golf ball injury.

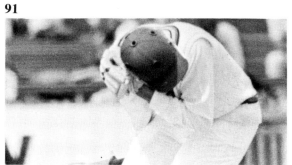

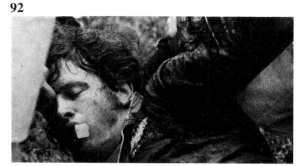

91 Even adequate headgear may not protect entirely from a blow on the head.

92 Severe concussion with unconsciousness will require vigorous resuscitation.

Even mild cases of concussion should be treated. The ten-second rule should apply in all sports.

After head injury supervised observation is mandatory. No player who has been concussed should be allowed home unaccompanied. Significant loss of consciousness demands proper hospitalisation and follow up. Return to sport should be gradual and delayed. The possibility of late sequelae, e.g. subdural haematoma, must never be forgotten.

Eye injury

Too many eye injuries occur in sport even when protection is worn. They vary in severity from the corneal abrasion or subconjunctival haemorrhage to disruption of the eye ball, and some are due to deliberate violence. All eye injuries should be regarded as serious and referred for specialist attention.

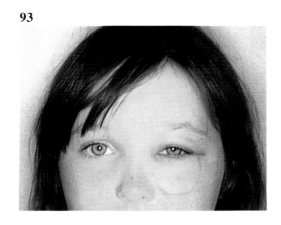

93 **Facial injury** due to blow from a tennis ball – the patient was wearing glasses.

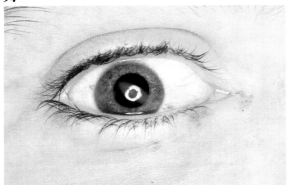

94 **Corneal abrasion** – stained with fluorescin dye.

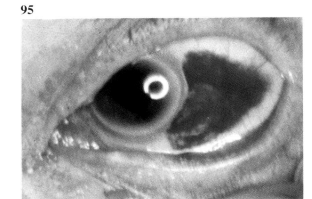

95 **Subconjunctival haemorrhage.** Looks dramatic but it is usually not serious.

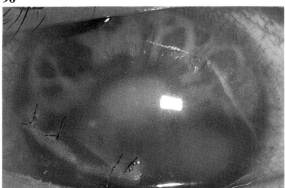

96 **Hyphaema.** Blood in the anterior chamber – a blow from a squash ball.

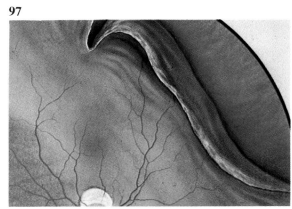

97 **Retinal detachment.** A real risk in the myope in body contact sport.

Facial injury

Injury to the face is mostly due to body contact sport, particularly in those events where face guards are not worn. As a rule, except in high-velocity vehicular injuries, damage is relatively slight, though the vulnerability of the eye, the teeth, and the jaw must not be forgotten. In sports involving implements or missiles, for example in ice hockey, lacrosse or cricket, facial protection may be necessary.

98

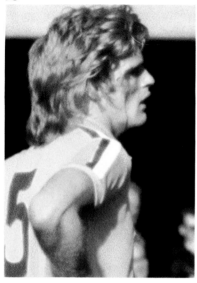

98 'Cut eye'. A supraorbital laceration in a footballer.

99

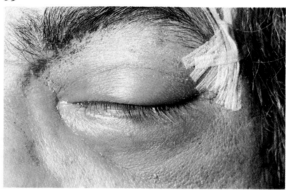

99 Haematoma of the eye (black-eye). This particular injury was associated with fractured zygoma.

100

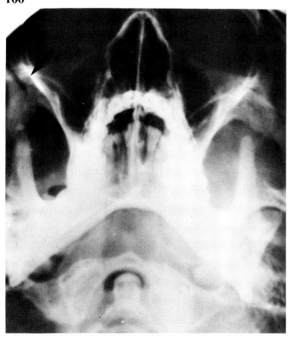

101

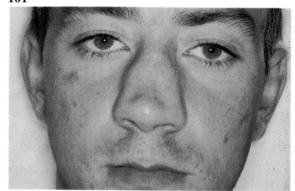

101 Fractured nasal bone. Almost invariably caused by combat body contact sports such as boxing or judo.

100 Fracture of zygoma. A not uncommon injury after a punch-up in rugby football.

102

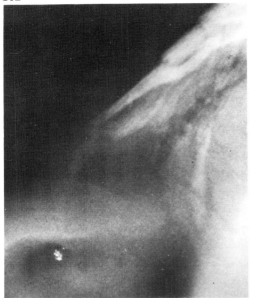

102   Radiograph of nasal fracture.

104

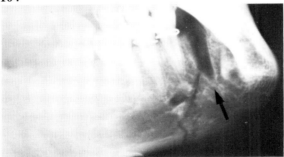

104   Radiograph of mandibular fracture. Note empty tooth socket.

106

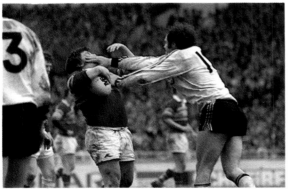

106   Facial injury. How it happens! Injury to the face is always a risk when the rules are forgotten and tempers lost.

103

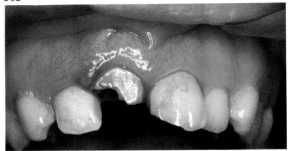

103   Dental injury. Teeth broken by direct violence. The wearing of mouth-guards will prevent such damage and is particularly recommended in rugby football and boxing.

105

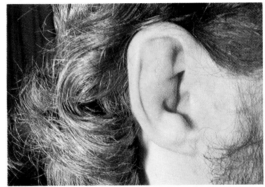

105   Haematoma of auricle – 'cauliflower ear'. In the acute phase evacuation of the haematoma and compression dressing may prevent the typical deformity of the ear. Protection is given by wearing a scrumcap or binding adhesive tape around the head to cover the ears.

107

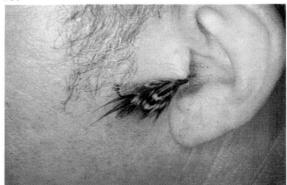

107   'Foul-hooked'!

5 Neck injuries

Cervical spine

Congenital abnormalities

Congenital abnormalities of the cervical spine are relatively unimportant and are often incidental findings. However, relative impairment of normal function produced by these conditions may be sufficient to interfere with sporting activity. Where some specific potential weakness is present, sport may be completely contraindicated.

108

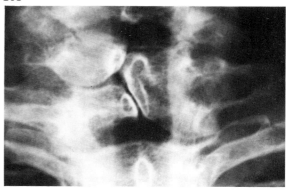

108 Cervical spina bifida occulta. An antero-posterior radiograph.

109

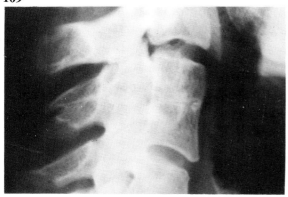

109 Congenital fusion of the 3rd and 4th cervical vertebra. A lateral radiograph.

110

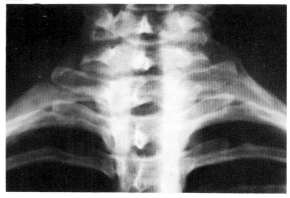

110 Cervical ribs. An anteroposterior radiograph. This condition is associated with interference with function of the distal root of the brachial plexus and the subclavian artery. It is this interference with function that brings the patient for treatment.

Patients presenting with cervical symptoms in whom these types of conditions are found should be cautioned away from neck-stressing sports, i.e. association and rugby football, trampolining and gymnastics, judo and wrestling.

Injuries

Fortunately injuries of the cervical spine are relatively uncommon, but because of the vulnerability of the spinal cord the consequences may be tragic. The nature of the danger situations must be recognised and where possible factors liable to cause injury, for example the spearing tackle in American football, must be banned. The possibility of cervical cord damage must always be remembered in patients sustaining neck injuries in sport, particularly body-contact sport. Where the possibility of such injuries is real, e.g. in rugby football, appropriate facilities must be available for adequate first aid and resuscitation if necessary.

Danger situations

111

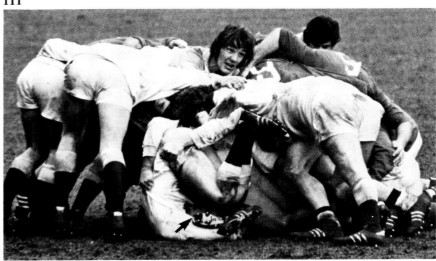

111 The rugby scrummage collapses. Note position of arrowed player.

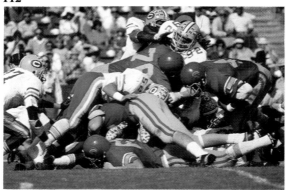

112 Multiple pile-up in the gridiron game.

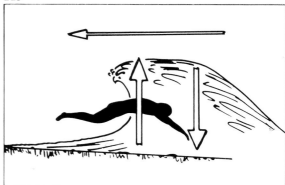

113 Diving into shallow water, particularly if the bottom cannot be seen easily.

In these examples as in other danger situations it is typically forced flexion with rotation (less commonly forced hyperextension) that does the damage. Rigid control by referees and self-control by players will reduce the hazard. Risk situations should if possible be removed from the sport, if necessary by changing the rules.

114

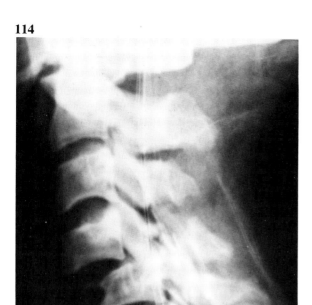

115

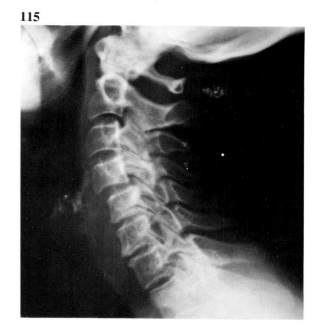

114 Dislocation. Lateral radiograph showing dislocation at C.4/5 (a diving accident). This type of injury is associated with gross neurological damage leading to tetraplegia.

115 Subluxation. Lateral radiograph showing subluxation at C.4/5 (a riding accident). This type of injury may be associated with transient neurological damage. The patient often complains of symptoms related to the local nerve roots.

Wedge fracture and subluxation – a rugby injury. Lateral radiographs taken during screening.

116

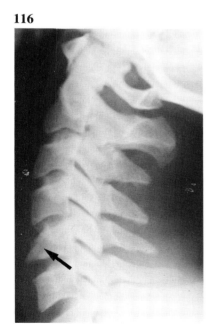

117

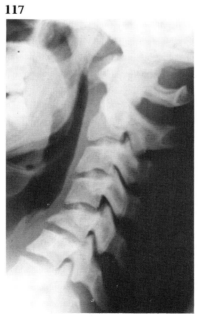

118

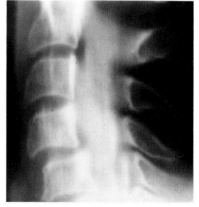

118 (In forced flexion) narrowing of spinal canal.

This patient, a teenage junior international, was experiencing minimal symptoms. Nevertheless, an injury of this type inevitably means a complete ban on further rugby football or other neck-stressing sports.

116 (In extension) deformity of C5 vertebral body.

117 (In flexion) forward subluxation of C4.

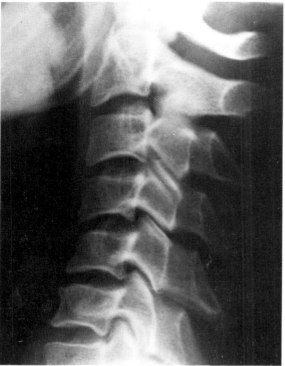

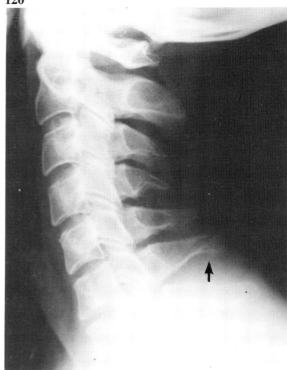

119 Loss of normal cervical contour due to muscle spasm (a rugby forward). Neurological signs are unusual, but root pain is commonly a symptom due to inflammation of the posterior facetal joints.

120 Fracture of spinous process of C6. A rugby-forward's injury due to *indirect* violence, the pull of the muscles on the ligament nuchae.

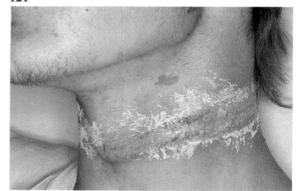

121 Rope burn on neck in motorcycle trialist running off circuit into boundary rope.

Happily in sport most spinal injuries are relatively minor, although occasionally and tragically severe injury with spinal cord damage occurs. Where causative factors can be clearly identified, for example in swimming (diving into shallow water) and in rugby football (deliberate collapsing of the scrum), every attempt should be made both by persuasion and coercion to eliminate dangerous activities. In all cases of doubt the possibility of spinal cord damage with its potential consequences must be remembered. The patient must be handled with utmost caution.

6 Shoulder and arm injuries

Clavicle

122

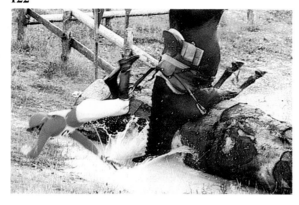

122 Fractures of the clavicle are common in sport, often associated with a fall; for example riding.

123

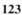

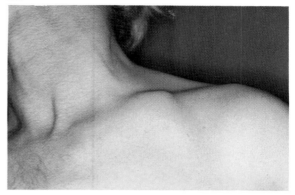

123 Typical appearance of clavicular fracture with obvious bone deformity.

124

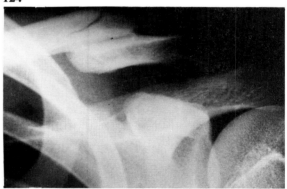

124 Refracture. Result of a young judoka returning to his sport too soon. Consolidation must be well advanced before sport is resumed, particularly if bone-end apposition is poor.

125

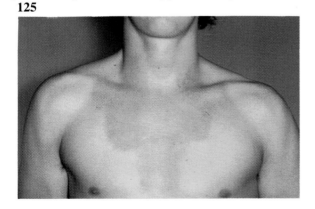

125 Sternoclavicular subluxation. Clinical appearance. A relatively unusual condition difficult to treat if the joint becomes clinically unstable.

126

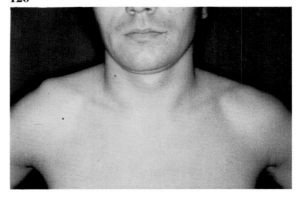

126 Acromioclavicular subluxation. Clinical appearance. A common injury due to a fall on the point of the shoulder. Note obvious deformity.

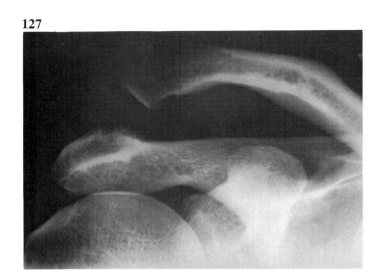

127 Acromioclavicular subluxation. Radiological appearance.

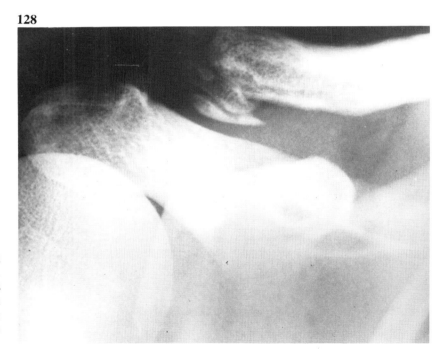

128 Ectopic calcification in acromioclavicular injury. Radiological appearance. This condition is associated with repeated capsular injury, in this case to a rugby league footballer.

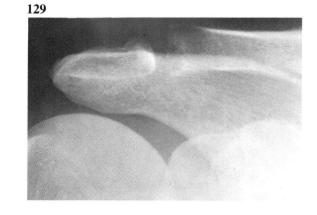

129 Traumatic osteolysis. Radiograph showing cystic appearance of outer end of clavicle in a patient sustaining repeated minor trauma of the acromioclavicular joint; in this case as the result of rugby football. This is probably the sequel to repeated articular cartilage damage whereas ectopic calcification (**128**) is associated with repeated capsular damage.

Scapula

Fractures of the scapula occur uncommonly in sport and are usually not serious, although frequently painful.

130 a

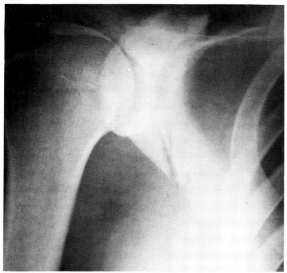

130a   Fracture of the wing of the scapula just medial to the glenoid in a young county rugby player.

130 b

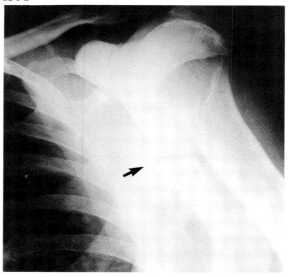

130b   Fracture of the whole blade of the scapula. Treatment of these injuries is essentially symptomatic with relief of pain and early mobilisation as the object.

131

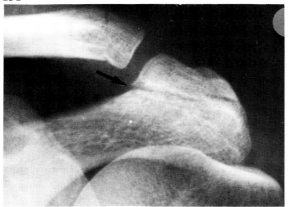

131   Fracture of the acromion in a footballer after a charge tackle. *Note:* There is a fracture of the outer end of the clavicle as well. In some views there may appear to be a fracture of the acromion, but this is an artefact due to projection, unless a break in the cortical margin is shown.

132

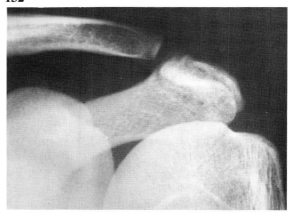

132   Acromial abnormality in a young javelin thrower; in this case an ununited ossification centre is present in the outer end of the acromion.

Shoulder joint

Shoulder joint injuries are particularly common in sport. They may be the result of overuse, as in racket games such as badminton and tennis, or as a result of throwing and bowling as in cricket. Alternatively they may occur by direct violence, either in body contact sport, such as rugby union and league football or as the result of a fall.

Generally the clinical picture is similar to shoulder injuries in other activities. Because the shoulder joint is so dependent on soft-tissues for its stability, injuries to these structures are common and tend to become chronic. Disability is often out of proportion to the extent of the tissue damage.

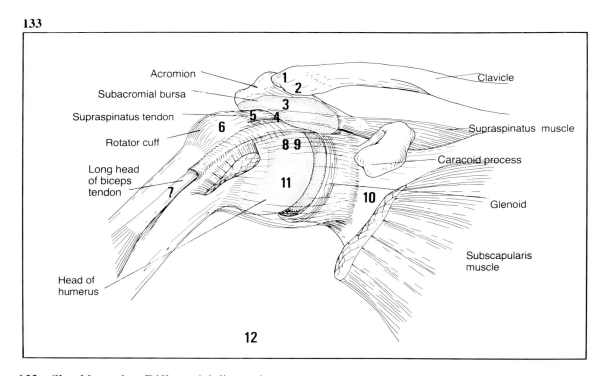

133 Shoulder pain. Differential diagnosis.

1 Acromioclavicular sprain/subluxation/dislocation/osteoarthrosis/bursitis
2 Traumatic osteolysis   lateral end of clavicle
3 Subacromial bursitis
4 Supraspinatus tendonitis
5 Supraspinatus } calcification rupture
6 Rotator cuff
7 Bicipital tendonitis
8 Capsulitis of shoulder joint
9 'Frozen shoulder'
10 Recurrent subluxation/dislocation
11 Osteoarthrosis
12 Referred pain

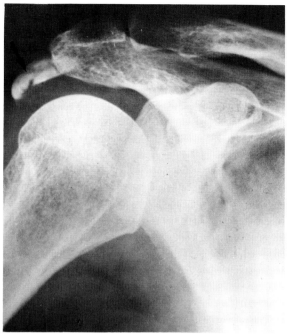

134 Ectopic calcification showing typical appearances of calcium deposit: supraspinatus tendon.

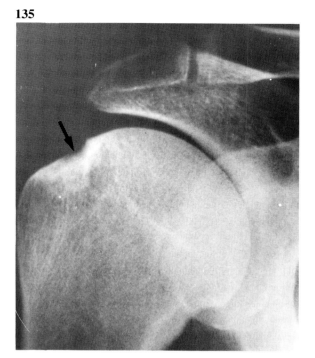

135 Rotator cuff injury showing erosion on greater tuberosity.

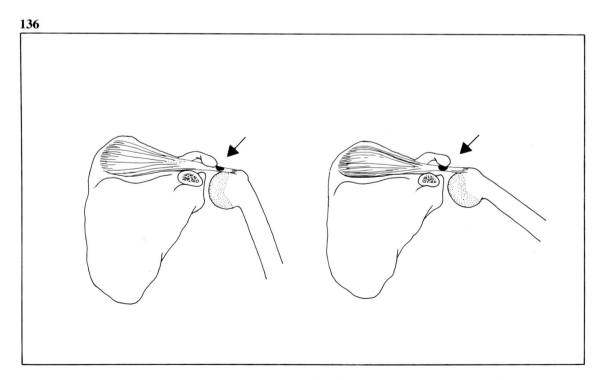

136 Supraspinatus tendonitis. Diagram showing production of symptoms in the painful arc.

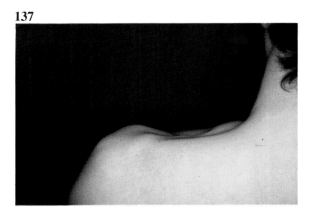

137 Bicipital tendonitis. Clinical photograph showing localised swelling over the anterior aspect of the shoulder due to inflammation and effusion into the biceps tendon sheath.

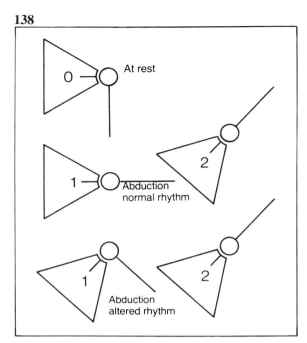

138 Scapulohumeral rhythm. Normal pattern with initial abduction at shoulder joint. Altered rhythm with abduction by rotation of scapula.

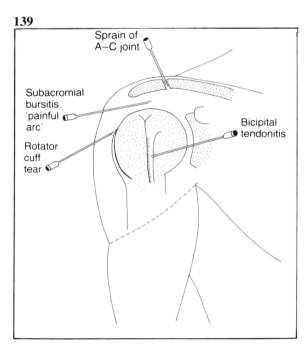

139 Diagram showing sites of injection for common causes of shoulder pain.

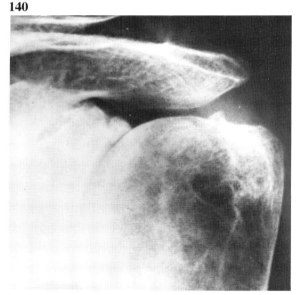

140 Degenerative disease. Osteoarthrosis of the shoulder joint. A rare condition often associated with a history of recurrent dislocation.

The management of shoulder injuries in sportsmen is similar to that for the population as a whole. Diffuse lesions such as capsulitis are best treated with systemic anti-inflammatory medication and physiotherapy (e.g. shortwave diathermy), while well-localised lesions usually respond well to local anaesthetic and steroid injection.

Dislocation

141

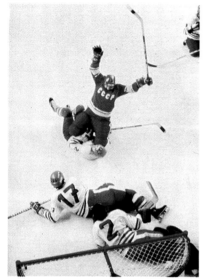

141 The common mechanism of dislocation. The arm is forcibly abducted and externally rotated, either in a fall or a 'pile-up', as in this ice hockey incident, giving anterior dislocation.

142

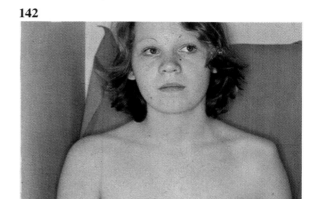

142 An anterior dislocation. Clinical appearance of the most common type.

143

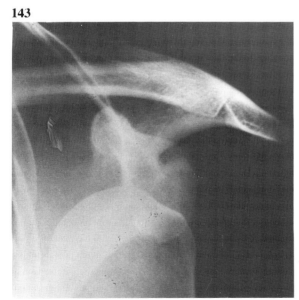

143 An anterior dislocation. Radiological appearance.

144

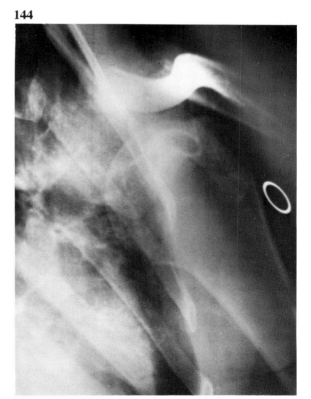

144 A posterior dislocation, much less common than an anterior dislocation. Radiological appearance.

47

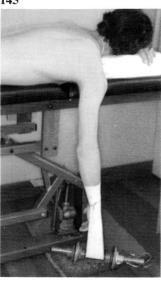

145   **Reduction of dislocation by Stimson method.** This is gentle manipulation and can be carried out immediately after dislocation. Note that the weight (in this case a dumbell) *hangs* on the arm and is not held by the patient. Reduction takes place with time as the patient relaxes.

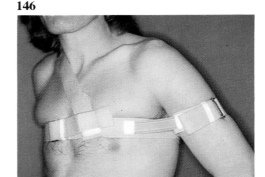

146   **Check rein** to allow movement of the shoulder (without abduction) during rehabilitation. Jockeys often return to the saddle early wearing such a device.

Injuries of the upper arm

Injuries of the upper arm are relatively unusual although a few examples are well known. They differ little from similar injuries sustained in non-sporting activity.

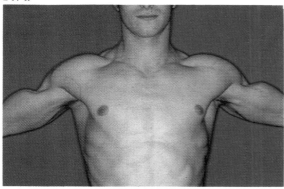

147a   **Bilateral rupture** of the long head of the biceps brachii in a gymnast. In this particular case the victim felt both tendons snap one after the other while exercising on the rings.

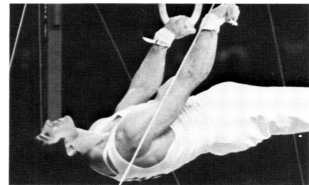

147b   **Defective biceps.** A gymnast competing internationally after subsequent rehabilitation. Defect in the biceps is clearly seen, and is of little functional significance.

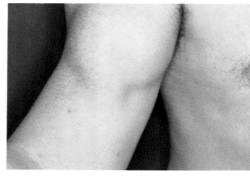

148   **Rupture of the biceps tendon** itself is less common than rupture of the tendon of the long head of the biceps.

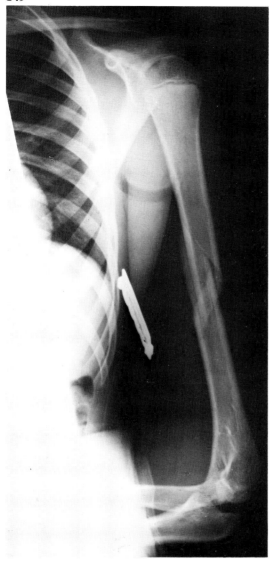

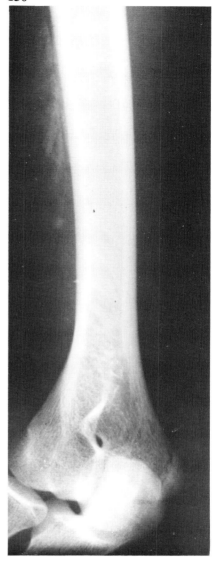

149 Gymnastic injury. Spiral fracture of the humerus as a result of fall from apparatus. Note that in this type of fracture radial-nerve involvement is common with wrist-drop and extensor weakness.

150 Myositis ossificans. A radiograph showing ectopic bone deposit in the brachialis on the anterior aspect of the humerus. Reabsorbed in six months.

Epiphysitis may occur at either end of the humerus in 'little league' and 'pitcher's arm' – these are overuse injuries which recover well with rest, provided the patient is not forced to play too soon after symptoms subside.

In some cases muscular violence may of itself be sufficient to cause fracture of humerus and spontaneous fracture has been described in a number of throwing accidents. It seems to be most common in baseball.

7 Elbow injuries

Congenital abnormalities

Mechanical abnormalities that may interfere with sport.

151

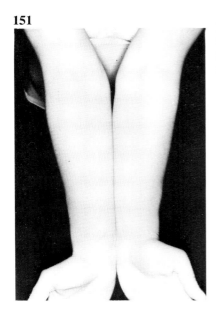

151 Cubitus valgus. This deformity predisposes to ulnar neuritis, particularly in throwers.

152

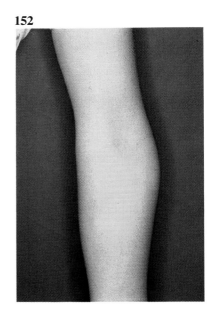

152 Cubitus varus. May be the result of an earlier supracondylar fracture. The joint is vulnerable in racquet games.

153

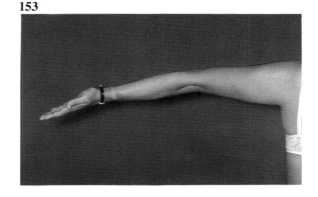

153 Cubitus recurvatus. Often a feature of hypermobile joint disease. Predisposes to olecranon impingement exostosis (see **165**).

Structural abnormalities of the elbow are commonly congenital although they may be acquired, usually as a result of an elbow fracture affecting the epiphyses during childhood which subsequently disturbs the normal growth of the lower end of the humerus. Cubitus valgus, varus and recurvatus may all cause problems, typically in sports involving throwing. Cubitus recurvatus may also cause problems in gymnastics.

Fractures and dislocations

Fractures about the elbow, as well as dislocations, require serious attention. Inadequate management, particularly in the early stages, may lead to permanent disability with disfigurement and loss of joint mobility. In dislocations and some fractures, particularly in children, the possibility of associated vascular and nerve damage must be remembered.

154

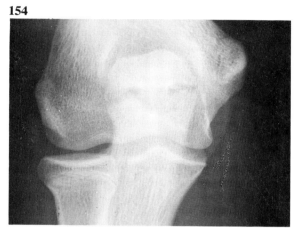

154   Fracture of the olecranon often due to indirect violence, i.e. violent contraction of triceps brachii.

155

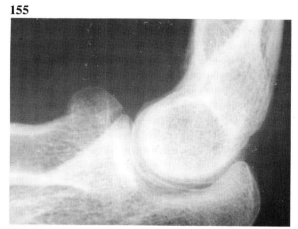

155   Fracture of radial head.   Radiograph. Resulted from a fall on the outstretched hand. If fragment is displaced some functional loss may follow.

156

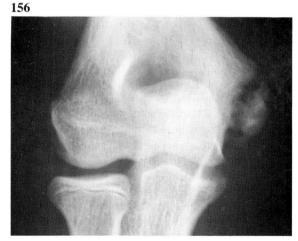

156   Avulsion of medial epicondyle. Radiograph. This type of injury is the result of indirect violence. The common flexor origin was pulled away in a gymnastic accident.

157

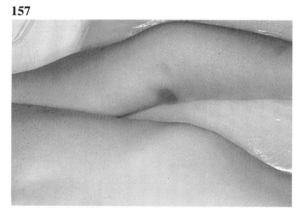

157   Dislocation of elbow.   Clinical appearance. This is usually the result of severe violence such as a fall from gymnastic apparatus.

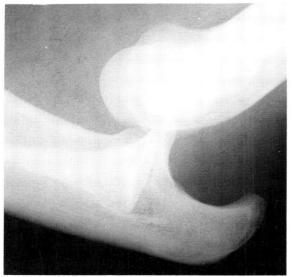

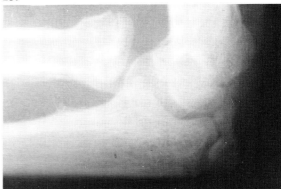

159   Old dislocation of superior radioulnar joint in a young gymnast. Radiograph. This exemplifies the tragic consequences of inadequate initial management. In this case particularly it was due to the failure to cope with the radial head dislocation.

158   Dislocation of elbow joint.   Radiograph.

Osteochondritis

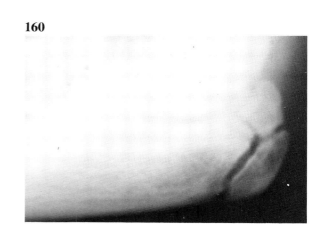

160   Osteochondritis of olecranon epiphysis in a young male tennis player (age 14). Radiograph. It is not clear whether this is a true traction epiphysitis caused by the pull on the triceps tendon, or whether there is an element of impingement injury resulting from repeated forced extension of the elbow joint.

161   Osteochondritis of capitellum in a young female gymnast (age 12) with loose body formation. Radiograph.

Both these cases illustrate the damage that can accrue to the joints of highly talented young sportsmen and women who are overstrained in training during their adolescent years.

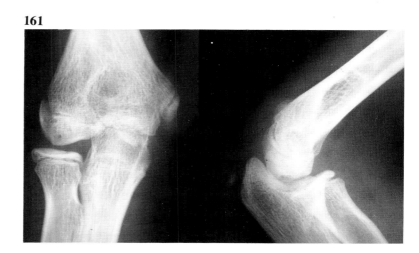

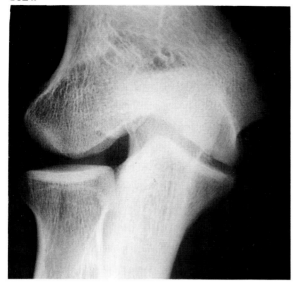

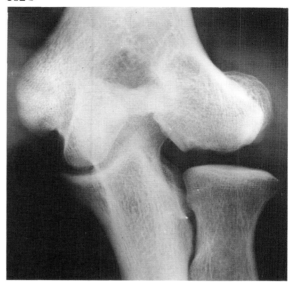

162a Limited extension. Radiograph of elbow joint in a young rugby player with limited extension. Probably congenital as the other elbow was identical (**162b**).

163

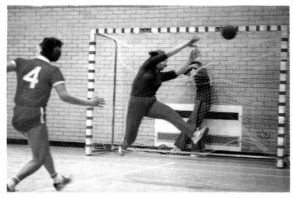

163 Handball. A sport demanding vigorous forward extension of the elbow.

164

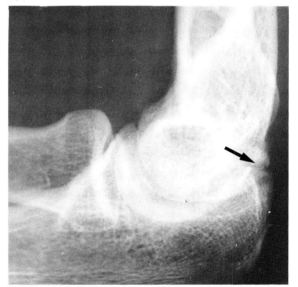

164 Loose bodies due to separation of impingement exostosis on tip of olecranon process of the ulna in an international handball player.

The exostosis develops as a result of repeated banging of the tip of the olecranon into its fossa during forced hyperextension.

Loose bodies

Loose bodies in the elbow, as elsewhere, may cause pain and discomfort related to their predisposing pathology and will also produce locking by interference with normal joint mechanism. In the latter case surgical removal is necessary but the long-term outcome is not necessarily good.

165

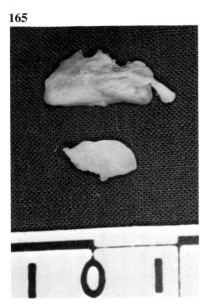

165 Specimen of loose body after surgical removal.

166

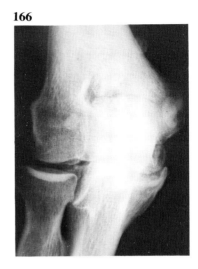

166 Loose bodies associated with degenerative joint disease in a squash player.

167

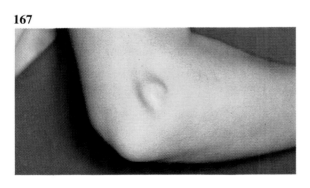

167 Ganglion over the lateral epicondyle. Something of a rarity.

168

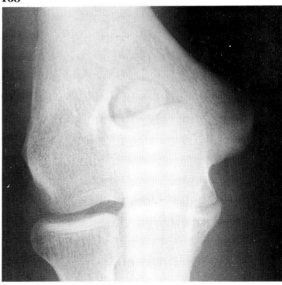

168 Olecranon fossa abnormality. Not a loose body! A congenital abnormality in the olecranon fossa of a cricketer (fast bowler). His inability to extend the elbow fully lead to his being frequently 'no-balled' (for chucking) when bowling.

169

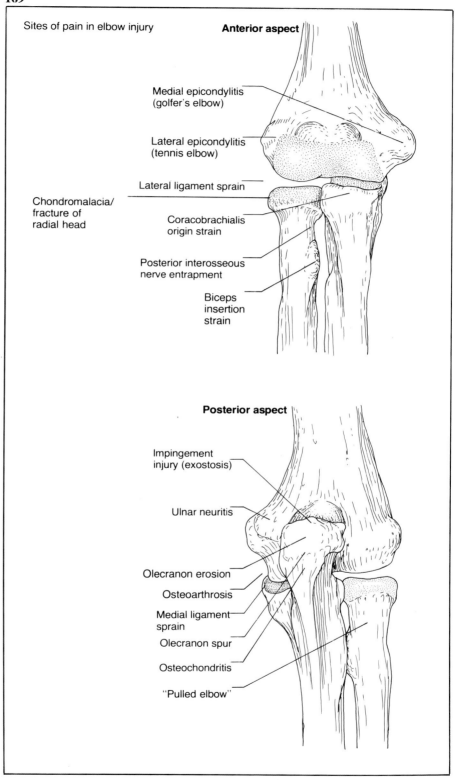

Sites of pain in elbow injury

Anterior aspect

Medial epicondylitis
(golfer's elbow)

Lateral epicondylitis
(tennis elbow)

Lateral ligament sprain

Chondromalacia/
fracture of
radial head

Coracobrachialis
origin strain

Posterior interosseous
nerve entrapment

Biceps
insertion
strain

Posterior aspect

Impingement
injury (exostosis)

Ulnar neuritis

Olecranon erosion

Osteoarthrosis

Medial ligament
sprain

Olecranon spur

Osteochondritis

"Pulled elbow"

169   Sites of pain. Differential diagnosis of elbow pain.

Lateral epicondylitis (tennis elbow)

Common causes of this condition include playing a whipped (topspin) backhand at tennis and using a badminton racket with too small a handle.

170

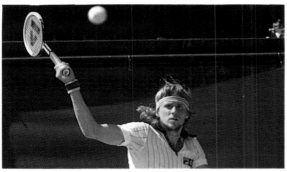

170 Topspin backhand. Note position of the racquet head in this international player applying heavy topspin.

171

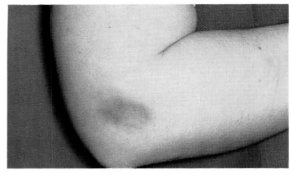

171 Lateral epicondylitis. Marked bruising over lateral epicondyle in recent acute tennis elbow.

172

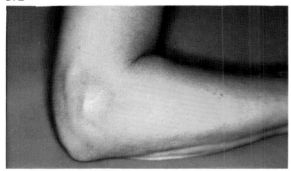

172 Skin change over lateral epicondyle as a result of previous hydrocortisone injection. Note discoloration of skin – this is associated with thinning of the dermis and loss of subcutaneous fat.

173

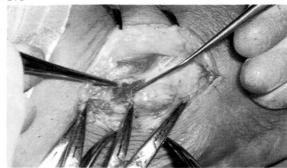

173 Surgical tenotomy of common extensor origin for tennis elbow. A radical method of treatment for recalcitrant chronic lesions.

174

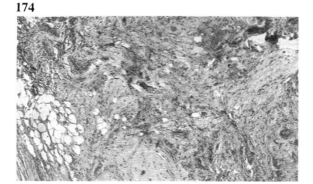

174 Scar tissue. Histological appearance of scar tissue removed at tenotomy showing completely random mixture of old and new scar tissue formation.

175

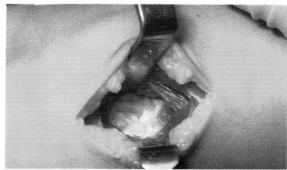

175 Posterior interosseous nerve entrapment. A cause of 'tennis elbow' symptoms. Appearance at operative decompression.

Golfer's elbow

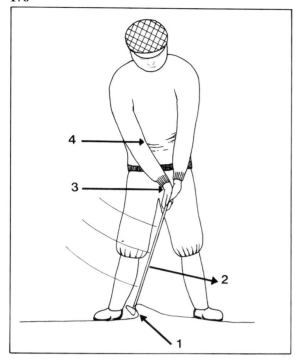

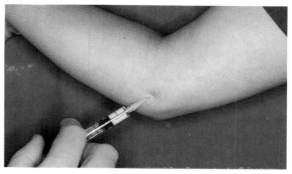

177 Medial epicondylitis. Golfer's elbow treated by local anaesthetic and steroid injection into the tender muscle attachment.

176 Common flexor origin. Club head blocked (**1**) causes forward rotation of shaft (**2**), forcibly hyperextending wrist (**3**), and pulling common flexor origin (**4**).

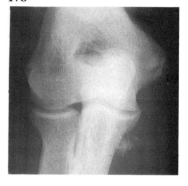

178 Calcification in common flexor mass. A radiograph. A late complication of recurrent golfer's elbow.

Thrower's elbow (medial collateral ligament sprain)

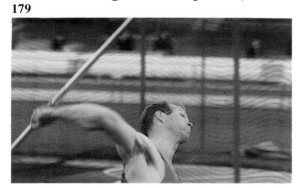

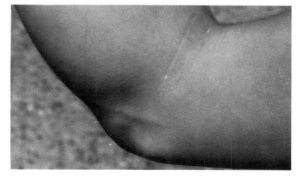

179 Mechanism of injury – the 'round arm' throw.

This condition should not be treated with local anaesthetic and steroid injection in view of the risk of subsequent laxity or rupture – an all too common complication at this site.

180 Clinical appearance with loss of normal common flexor muscle bulk.

Pulled elbow

Subluxation of radial head in children. This is a condition in which the head of the radius is pulled out of the annular ligament as a result of traction on the arm. It occurs in body-contact sports including judo. Associated fractures are uncommon and usually self-evident.

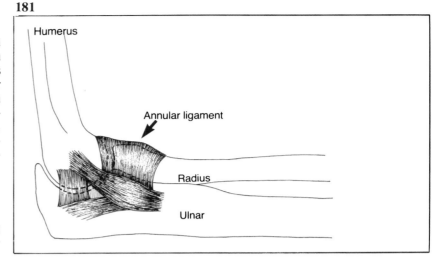

181 Diagram showing normal anatomy of annular ligament and pulled elbow.

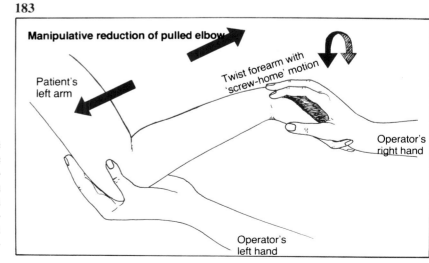

182 Mechanism of pulled elbow.

183 Manipulation. Reduce with the elbow at right angle by a rotary screwing movement of alternate pronation and supination of forearm while pushing the radius towards the elbow. Reduction is easily achieved, accompanied by a palpable 'click'.

Elbow joint – degenerative change

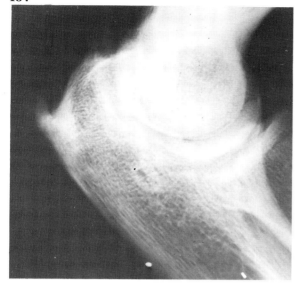

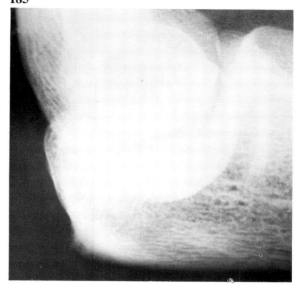

184 Spur on tip of olecranon at triceps insertion in tennis player.

185 Erosion on tip of olecranon at triceps insertion in international fencer.

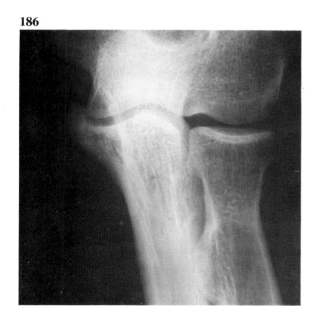

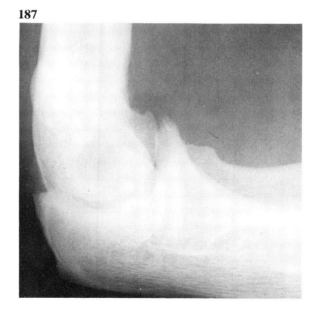

186 Spur on ulna in squash player.

187 Spur on coronoid process in badminton player.

Unless causing localised symptoms these lesions may be left undisturbed. When causing symptoms conservative treatment (e.g. local anaesthetic and steroid injection) may be inadequate, particularly if there is any mechanical disturbance, in which case surgical removal may be required.

8 Forearm, wrist and hand injuries

Tenosynovitis of the extensor tendons of the wrist

188

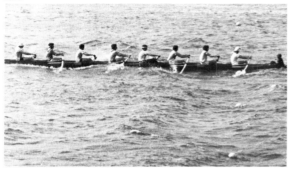

189

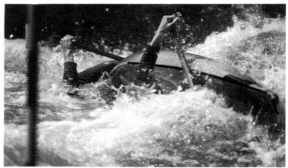

188 and 189 Tenosynovitis. This condition is common in oarsmen and canoeists, often associated with training in rough water.

190

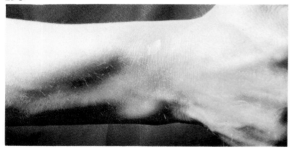

190 Tenosynovitis. The clinical picture is of swelling and crepitus on the dorsum of the forearm.

191

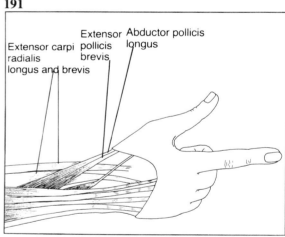

191 Anatomy of the abductor pollicis longus and the extensor pollicis brevis overlying the radial extensors of the wrist. The muscle bellies are frequently hypertrophied and oedematous in this condition with adhesion to the underlying tissues.

192

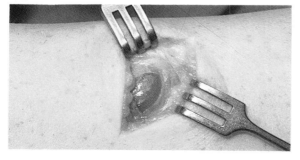

192 Surgical decompression of abductor pollicis longus and extensor pollicis brevis muscles gives early and effective relief, as the muscle bulges up through the incision in the sheath relieving pressure on the tendons beneath. Return to normal function is possible within a matter of hours.

Wrist injuries

Wrist injuries are relatively uncommon, but may be a source of considerable disability. Fractures and sprains are no different from those incurred in normal activities, but impingement lesions, as for example in 'thrower's wrist', are not commonly met outside sport.

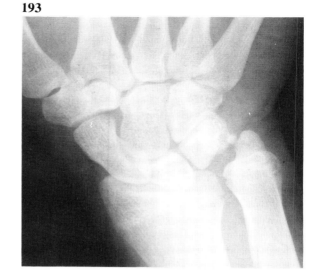

193   Congenital abnormality. Prominence of the ulnar styloid associated with a chip fracture. This patient complained of inability to push the hand into ulnar deviation together with pain while playing racket games.

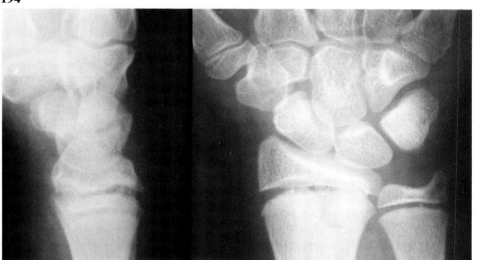

194   Epiphysiolysis without displacement in young gymnast. Note appearance of epiphysial line. This condition should be treated as a fracture and immobilised.

195   Epiphysiolysis with displacement in footballer.

In some cases of persistent wrist pain associated with an apparent chronic sprain stress xrays in radial and ulnar deviation may demonstrate traumatic diastasis of the scaphoid from the lunate.

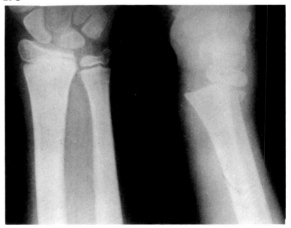

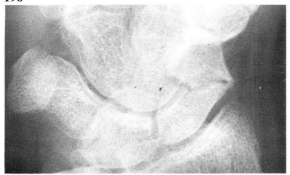

196 Radiograph of ununited fracture of the scaphoid. This injury commonly occurs in a fall on an outstretched hand and may be undetected in the early stages. Early diagnosis and effective immobilisation obviates the risk of non-union and later osteoarthrosis.

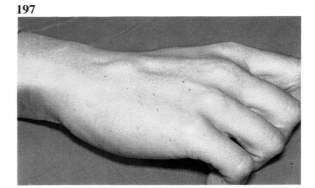

197 Thrower's wrist. Prominence of the styloid process of the 2nd or 3rd metacarpals may cause nipping of the soft tissues in the hyperextension of the wrist.

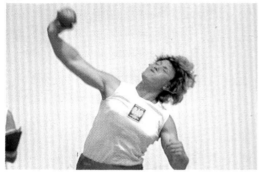

198 Thrower's wrist: hyperextension. Putting the shot: note marked hyperextension of the wrist as the athlete accelerates the shot in the action of projecting it.

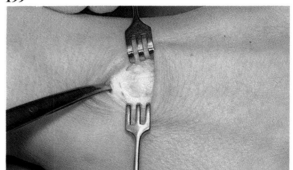

199 Thrower's wrist: treatment. In chronic resistant cases treatment is excision of the underlying boss of bone.

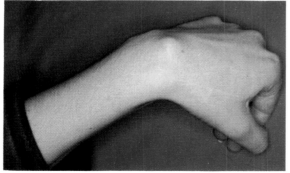

200 A ganglion. Soft-tissue swelling on the dorsum of the wrist. A common problem.

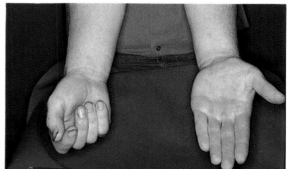

201 Interosseous nerve palsy. A real oddity. Posterior interosseous nerve palsy in a tyro – water skier. A traction injury.

Radiocarpal joint injury

Injury to the distal radioulnar joint is an occasional source of disability. Interference with pronation and supination may be due to loose body or dislocation of the triangular meniscus and will often require surgical exploration.

Thumb injuries

Thumb injuries are most common in boxing.

202

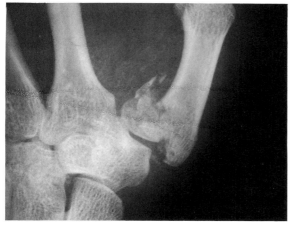

202 Bennett's fracture. Fracture of the base of the 1st metacarpal through the joint line.

203

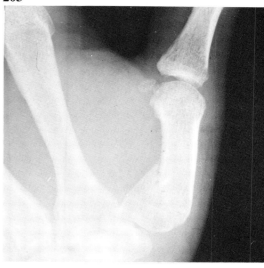

203 Fracture of the base of the 1st metacarpal with no joint involvement.

204

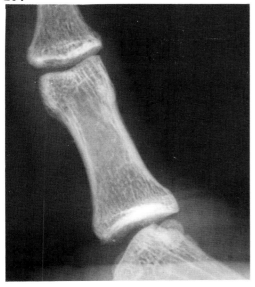

204 Dislocation of the thumb associated with rupture of the ulnar collateral ligament in an Olympic medallist (otherwise known as 'game-keeper's thumb').

205

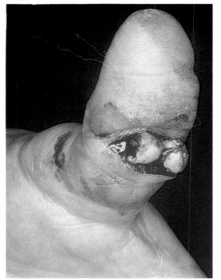

205 Compound dislocation of the thumb. For a change, a rugby injury!

206

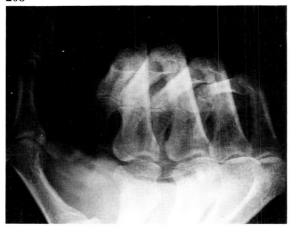

207

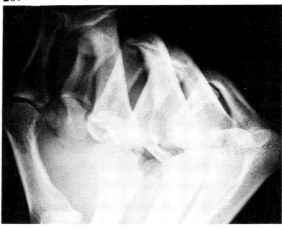

206 Radiograph of a fist clenched within boxing glove showing vulnerability of thumb.

207 Ungloved fist for comparison.

An occasional problem in boxing is thickening of the metacarpophalangeal joint due to repeated fracture ('boxer's knuckle') often associated with damage to intermetacarpal ligament. A metacarpophalangeal bursitis is also described.

Finger injuries

These injuries are common in body-contact sports, hard ball games (particularly cricket), and in judo (which involves grasping the opponent's clothing).

208 a

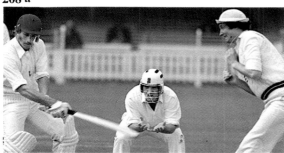

208 b

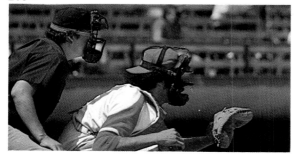

209

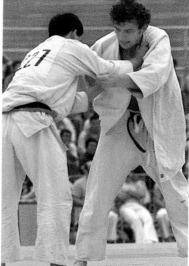

208a Fingers are at risk in any catching game, particularly cricket. **b** Some protection is obtained by wearing suitably padded gloves – baseball catcher.

209 In judo finger damage occurs when holds on the opponent's clothing are forcibly broken.

Finger fractures from sport

210

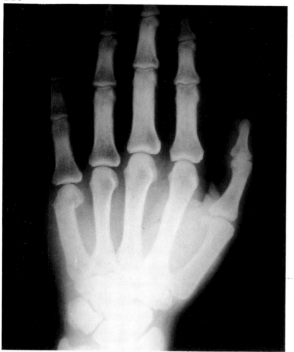

211

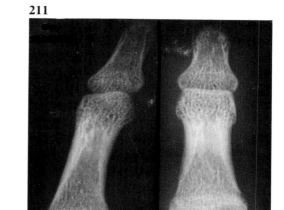

210 Metacarpal fracture. These are often self inflicted when the patient engages in rough play in body-contact sport and punches an opponent.

211 Proximal phalangeal fracture can occur when the hand grasping an implement, e.g. a hockey stick, is struck directly by a hard ball.

212

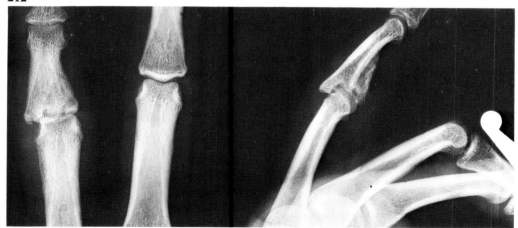

212 Fracture of the middle phalanx is relatively uncommon and, like that of the proximal, often caused by a blow from a ball, in this case from a cricket ball.

213 Terminal phalangeal fractures are very common not only in hard-ball games but also in basketball, volleyball and handball. In some cases, particularly with a direct blow in the long axis of the phalanx, the fracture line goes through the bone with disruption of the distal interphalangeal joint.

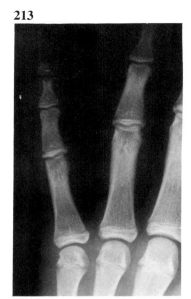
213

Other common finger injuries include interphalangeal subluxation or dislocation, subungual haematoma, avulsion of the nail and lacerations. They are no different from similar injuries incurred in non-sporting situations. In all cases the object of treatment is the early healing of the specific injury and vigorous rehabilitation from the earliest possible stage to secure maximum function.

214

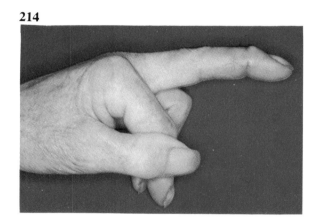

214 Mallet finger. Rupture of extensor tendon or avulsion of attachment due to a blow on the tip of the finger, as in slip fielding in cricket.

215

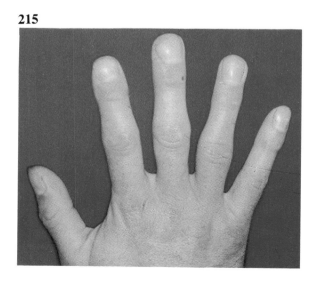

215 Old dislocation. Result of repeated injury in a judoka. Functional deformity is always preferable to loss of function of a cosmetically pleasing hand.

9　Trunk and abdominal injuries

Trunk injury

Most trunk injuries involve the musculoskeletal system of the spine and limb roots. Thoracic cage injuries are also quite common and the ever-present possibility of rib fracture being associated with underlying visceral damage must be borne in mind.

216

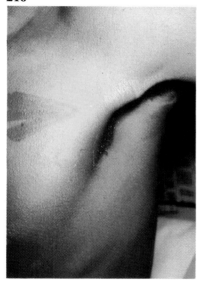

217

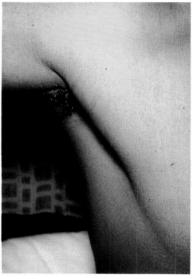

216 and 217 Rupture of pectoralis major with opposite side for comparison. This is an unusual injury. There is only one case of bilateral ruptured pectoralis major recorded in the literature.

218

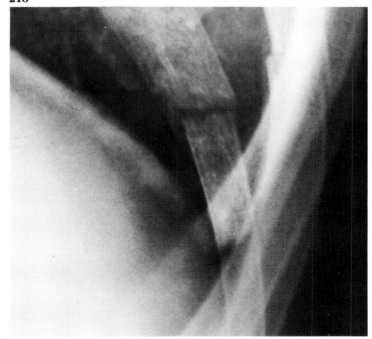

218 Rib fractures are common in rugby football and riding accidents. However, they may also occur as the result of a direct blow in any sport.

219

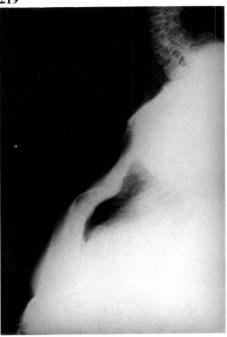

220

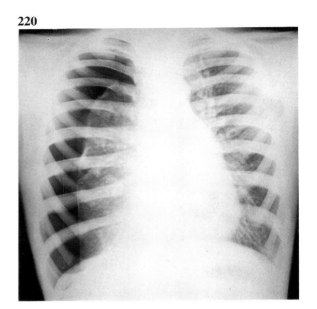

220 Pneumothorax associated with rib fracture. Radiological appearance.

219 Sternal fracture. A less common injury and usually the sequel of a vehicular injury.

221

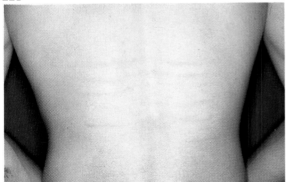

222

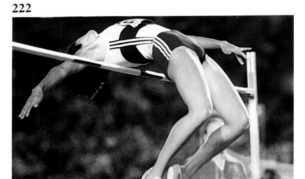

221 and 222 Weals on the back of an athlete. These lesions are not due to chastisement. The patient was a high jumper practising the Fosbury flop, repeatedly falling onto the landing area with the bar beneath him.

Other problems of trunk pathology may affect sports participation often because they cause concern on the part of the patient rather than from any immediate clinical reason. Congenital abnormalities may look disfiguring but are usually of little functional significance.

223

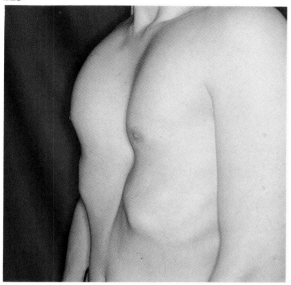

223 Pectus excavatus. A congenital abnormality of the chest. This patient was able to resume vigorous sporting activity after surgery to restore the normal contour of the sternum.

224

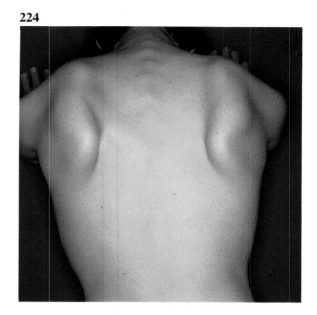

224 Winged scapulae. This patient was an international swimmer disabled as a result of neuralgic amyotrophy from a virus infection. He subsequently recovered completely to win an Olympic medal.

225a

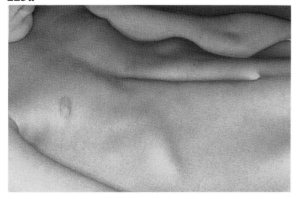

225b

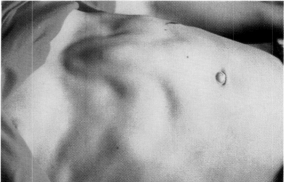

225a and b Defects in the linea alba. Congenital abnormalities in young football players. A matter of academic rather than clinical importance!

Abdominal injury

Soft tissue injury to the abdominal and pelvic viscera is rare in sport. When it occurs it is often associated with high velocity impact accidents (or occasionally with deliberate violence).

226

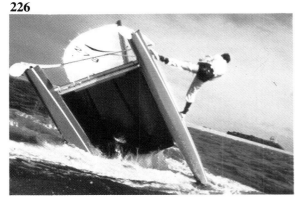

226 Abdominal injury occurs in high-velocity impacts (water can be very unyielding).

227

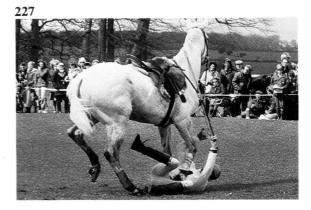

227 Abdominal injury also occurs in direct violence.

228

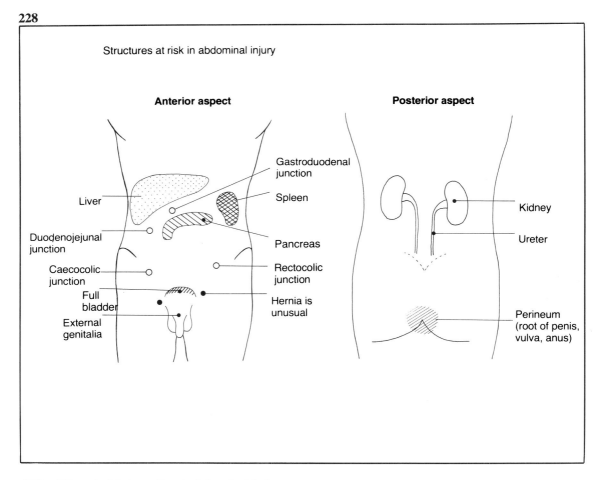

228 Sites at risk in a direct abdominal injury.

In the abdomen the structures at risk include liver, spleen and pancreas, together with the bowel, particularly when it becomes retroperitoneal. Thus the gastroduodenal and duodenojejunal junctions are particularly at risk. The large bowel is much more rarely involved in accidents of this type but it may be involved in penetrating injuries.

The genitourinary tract is also vulnerable, the kidneys to a blow in the loin and the bladder (particularly if full) and urethra to a blow in the lower abdomen and perineum.

An interesting form of orchitis has been described in youngsters going for early morning runs before emptying their bladders. Male external genitalia should always be protected at least by a supporter or jockey briefs and in hard-ball games such as cricket and hockey by a properly constructed box.

229

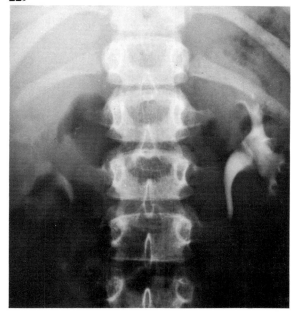

229 Intravenous pyelogram showing damage to right kidney.

230

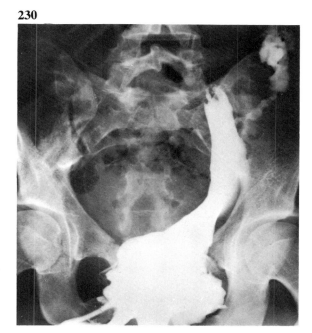

230 Cystogram showing extravasation of blood caused by rupture of the bladder.

232

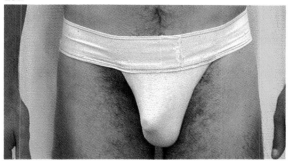

232 Wearing an athletic supporter or jockstrap reduces the risk of injury.

231

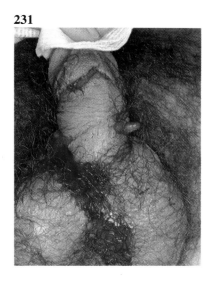

231 Genital injuries also occur in sport. Lacerations of the penis from a direct kick in a football accident.

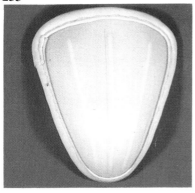

233 Protective gear. A box often worn by hockey players and cricketers. Not only should batsmen wear them, but also close-in fielders, especially those in the 'silly' positions.

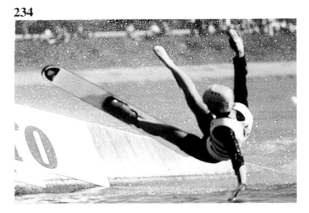

234 Water-skiing accident. In such instances water under pressure may be forced into the vagina (and even into the rectum) if adequate protective clothing is not worn.

The female genitalia are less vulnerable, as might be expected, but water-skiing presents particular problems of the high-pressure douche from an awkward fall. Adequate protection must be worn for serious competition and training.

Acquired hernia or rupture is unusual in sportsmen, probably because the well-developed abdominal muscles in the sportsman protect vulnerable sites.

Injuries to the abdominal wall are relatively uncommon and typically involve contusions from direct blows and muscle tears from intrinsic violence.

In all cases of abdominal injury the risk of visceral damage must be remembered, particularly if any form of direct violence is involved. Patients should be kept under strict observation and admit-ted to hospital if there is any deterioration in their condition. The ever-present risk of misdiagnosing the silent abdomen must be remembered and the patient observed at repeated intervals after a direct blow on the abdomen, before he can be regarded as being safe.

Spontaneous bleeding either as haematuria or haemoglobinuria is an occasional feature in high performance sport. The exact cause is uncertain. In some instances it results from damage to the red corpuscles in the active tissues, in some it is due to altered glomerular filtration dynamics and some instances of haematuria may be caused by trigonitis. The presence of blood in the urine should always be investigated; such investigation must be regarded as urgent if this symptom is associated with direct trauma.

10 Spinal injuries

Dorsal spine

Being well buttressed by the ribs, spinal injuries at this level are unusual except in severe riding and vehicular accidents, in which very heavy loads, often with a rotary component, are applied. Fractures tend to occur at the upper or lower end of the dorsal spine. The spinous processes give more protection from D4 to D8.

Soft tissue injuries are quite common as are intervertebral joint conditions including the 'locked facet' syndrome and the 'dorsal disc' syndrome with referred pain along an intercostal nerve. Osteochondritis (adolescent kyphosis), quite commonly interferes with sport.

236

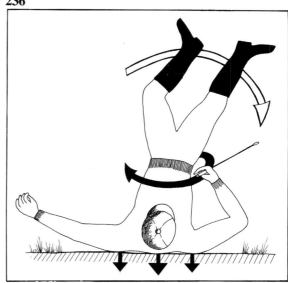

235

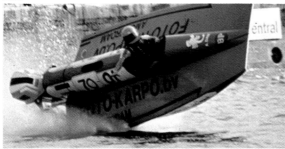

235 High speed vehicular accidents are a common cause of spinal injury.

236 Injury to the dorsal spine is typically the result of a combination of flexion compression and rotation stress.

237

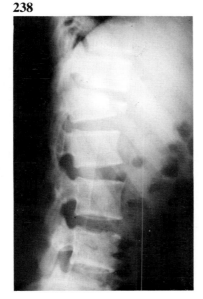

237 Upper dorsal spinal fracture.

238

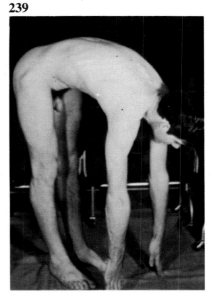

238 Lower dorsal spinal fracture.

239

239 Osteochondritis (adolescent kyphosis): loss of normal spinal contour.

Lumbar spine: congenital abnormality

These congenital abnormalities are a source of weakness in the spine which may be productive of symptoms in a patient undergoing heavy weight training and exercise programmes. The problem is essentially mechanical, usually associated with distortion of the intervertebral joint surfaces. These are generally a contraindication to such activities as weight lifting, rowing and athletic throwing events.

240

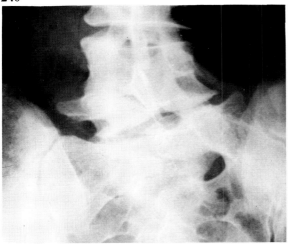

240 Hemivertebra. An anteroposterior radiograph.

241

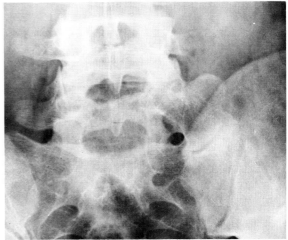

241 Sacralisation. Anteroposterior radiograph showing partial sacralisation (left side) of the 5th lumbar vertebra.

242

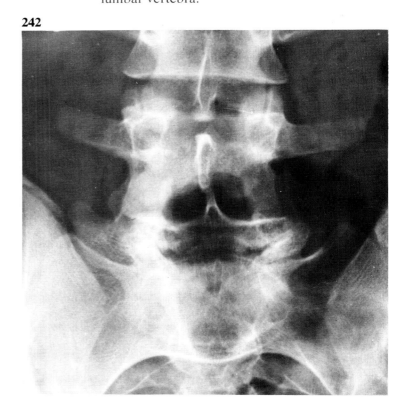

242 Partial lumbarisation of the 1st sacral vertebra. An anteroposterior radiograph.

In these conditions spinal stresses are transmitted asymmetrically and so introduce abnormal torque effects.

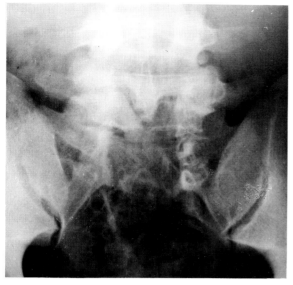

243 Spina-bifida occulta with distortion of the posterior facetal joints. An anteroposterior radiograph.

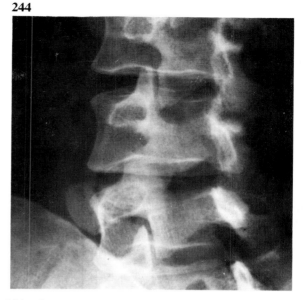

244 Posterior facetal joint. Oblique radiograph showing apparent loss of posterior facetal joint L4/5.

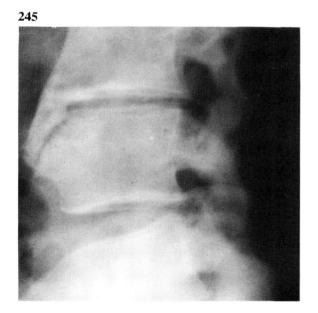

245 Lumbar vertebra. Abnormal ossification limbus vertebra.

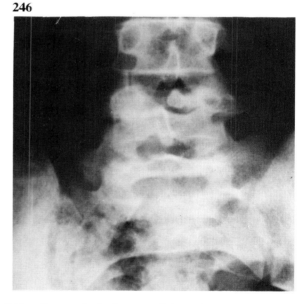

246 Congenital abnormalities. Anteroposterior radiograph showing congenital abnormalities of L5 and S1.

These abnormalities impede normal spinal mobility.

Most congenital spinal abnormalities are of relatively little clinical significance. Spina bifida has obvious clinical importance but the mild occult cases seldom cause problems. However, in in-dividuals engaged in high-performance activities the presence of spinal abnormalities may inter-fere with normal mechanical function and so provide a source of weakness.

Lumbosacral strain

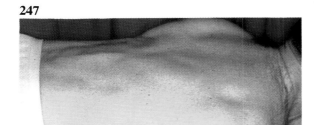

247 Spasm of the paravertebral muscles inhibiting extension, with loss of normal lumbar lordosis.

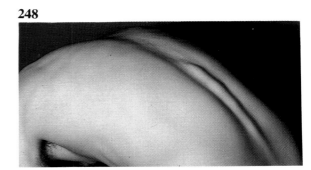

248 Spasm of the paravertebral muscles inhibiting flexion showing loss of normal prominence of spinous processes.

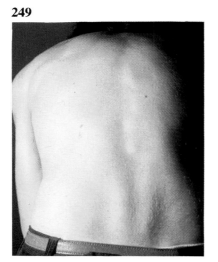

249 Spasm of paravertebral muscles causing scoliosis.

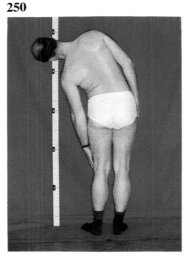

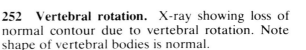

250 and 251 Asymmetry in lateral flexion due to unilateral spasm of paravertebral muscles.

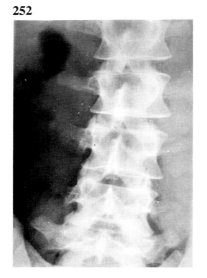

252 Vertebral rotation. X-ray showing loss of normal contour due to vertebral rotation. Note shape of vertebral bodies is normal.

Acute lumbosacral strain associated with spasm and limitation of movement, but no sciatic pain or neurological involvement.

Abnormal spinal curvature and loss of mobility are important signs of local muscle spasm. Restoration of normal mobility using spasmolytic drugs, ice or heat, traction manipulation and exercise is essential to secure relief of symptoms.

Ligament injuries

Ligament injuries such as sprung-back and kissing spine syndrome (hyperflexion and hyperextension injuries) seem quite rare in sport, except perhaps in diving and trampoline accidents. Usually the sportsman is fit enough to ride the stresses involved and only becomes injured with more severe stress, which tends to produce more severe injuries such as wedge fractures.

Overload injuries

Loading of the spine is quite severe in some training programmes and weight-training (as opposed to weight-lifting) is a potent cause of stress injury.

253

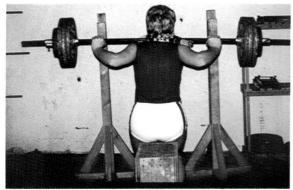

253 Lumbar spinal stress. Weight-training – a potent cause of lumbar spinal stress leading to stress fracture. Load is indicated by bend in bar (315lb) handled by this female athlete.

254

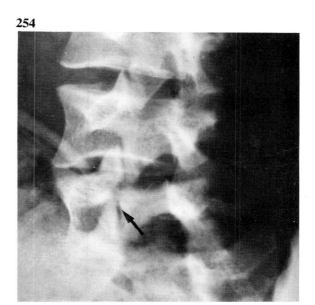

254 Spondylolysis. Stress fracture of the pars-interarticularis of L5 showing typical 'Scottie-dog with collar' appearance on oblique x-ray.

255

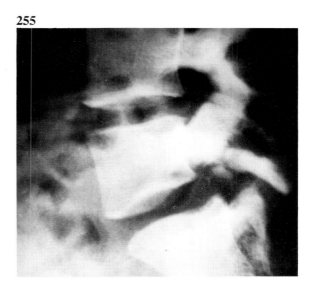

255 Spondylolysis in a tennis player. Lateral radiograph.
Treatment is by immobilisation to allow healing. Non-union may require immobilisation, but a re-markable number of patients seem to retain their fractures but lose their symptoms, perhaps because of fibrous rather than bony union.

Spondylolisthesis represents spinal instability and sport, particularly at a high level, is often impossible.

Even after successful surgery to stabilise the spine, caution dictates some restriction in activity.

256

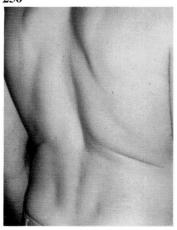

257

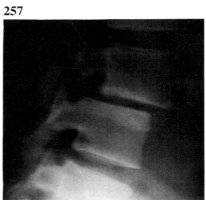

257 Radiograph showing forward slip (case 256).

256 Spondylolisthesis. Clinical photograph showing typical step in the lumbar spine of an international oarsman.

258

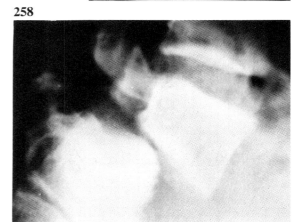

258 Radiograph of L5/S1 spondylolisthesis with marked displacement. This patient presented with a discomfort in the thigh while running and was diagnosed previously as a chronic hamstring strain.

259

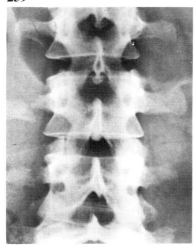

259 Fracture of transverse process due to a fall from a horse. Such fractures are occasionally due to muscle violence. In extrinsic injury the possibility of associated renal damage must be remembered.

260

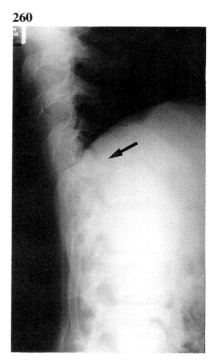

260 Spinal fracture associated with severe violence producing instability and spinal cord injury. A catastrophe, and the antithesis of all that sport intends.

Disc lesions

Disc lesions of the spine are difficult to diagnose clinically unless clearcut criteria are accepted. It is useful to restrict this term to those conditions where there is objective evidence of neurological disturbance associated with backache and referred pain in the legs. Almost invariably in these cases, particularly in the more chronic ones, evidence of disc prolapse will be demonstrable on contrast radiography.

261

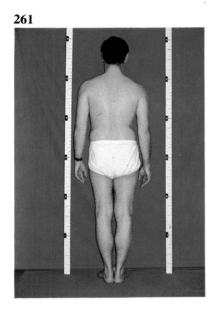

261 Typical sciatic scoliosis (associated with a disc lesion with loss of straight leg raising and neurological disturbance). Clinical photograph.

262

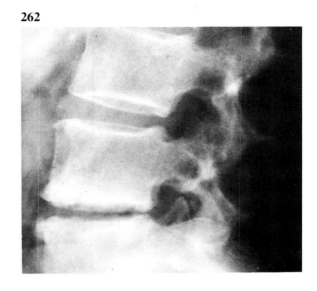

262 Radiograph showing disc degeneration at L4/5.

263

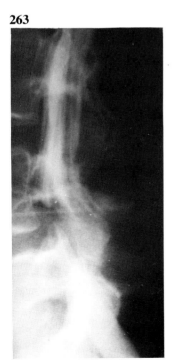

263 Disc protrusion. Lateral view of metrizamide radiculogram showing typical appearances of disc protrusion with filling defect.

264 Disc protrusion. Oblique view of myelogram showing typical disc protrusion.

If disc protrusions fail to settle rapidly exploration and removal of the prolapse is required. Return to sport should be gradual thereafter.

264

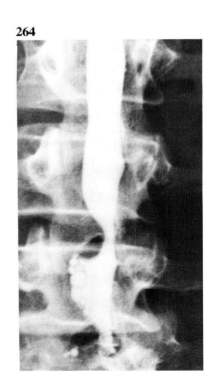

Spinal osteochondritis

True 'growing pains' are often associated with excessive training, particularly weight training.

The changes of osteochondritis are seen as much in the dorsal as in the lumbar spine; indeed in Scheuermann's disease the kyphosis may be the most immediately obvious factor although many patients with this condition complain of low back pain. The main significance of the osteochondritides is that in addition to causing pain in adolescence while the disease is active the subsequent distortion of the vertebral bodies, particularly where the patient is allowed to continue a rigorous sporting life, may predispose to degenerative joint disease at a later date.

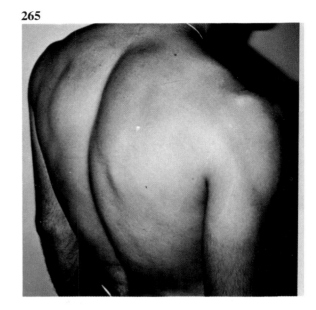

265

265 Scheuermann's disease. Clinical photograph showing dorsal kyphosis.

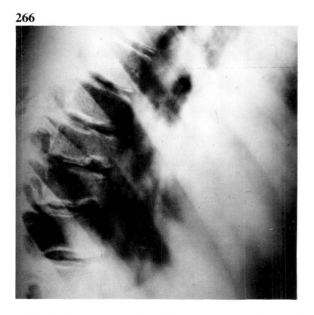

266

266 Scheuermann's disease. Radiological appearance.

267

267 Not osteochondritis. A congenital anomaly, a limbus vertebra.

Management is symptomatic, as the condition usually resolves with time.

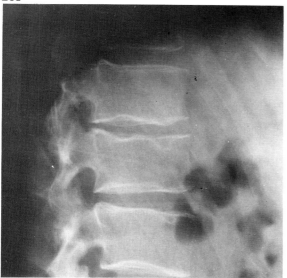

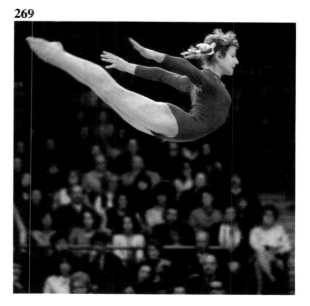

268   Osteochondritis. Lateral radiograph of adult spine showing distortion of vertebral bodies due to old osteochondritis.

269   Osteochondritis. Gymnastic agility – hyper-extension of the spine appears to be a common cause of osteochondritis and stress fractures of the spine in young girls.

Many of these conditions appear to be exacerbated by excessive load bearing in youth either due to over-vigorous attempts at mobilisation (for example in gymnastic training) or to the too early acceptance by the victims of heavy weight-training programmes. Generally it is advisable that loads exceeding the bodyweight should not be accepted as part of a weight-training programme until after skeletal maturity.

Sacrum and coccyx

These structures are almost injury free in sport. Injury to the sacroiliac joint may occur in severe pelvic damage, and a genuine sacroiliac strain may be associated with traumatic osteitis pubis.

While injuries to the sacrum and coccyx are relatively uncommon except in cases of direct violence, damage to the sacroiliac joint is often described although this may be a misinterpretation of strain of the insertion of erector spinae at the lower end over the sacroiliac joint. Ankylosing spondylitis, however, may present as an apparent sacroiliac injury caused by sport.

11 Pelvis and hip injuries

Pelvic injuries are quite common but usually mild being typically of the muscle origin/insertion avulsion type. More severe injury associated with direct violence occasionally occurs in vehicular accidents.

Os innominatum

270

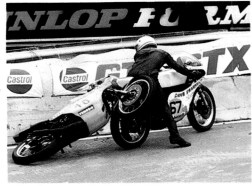

270 Major pelvic injury occurs in high-velocity impacts, as in motorcycle race crashes.

271

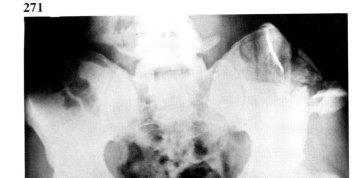

271 Major fracture due to direct violence. This type of injury occurs in riding and motor racing accidents.

272

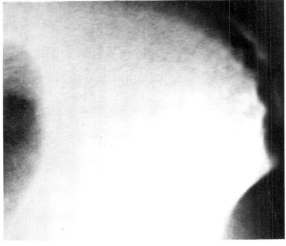

272 Avulsion of the iliac crest epiphysis. A stress injury in a young gymnast. Treatment is rest.

273

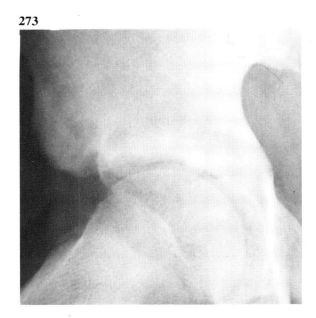

273 Avulsion injury of rectus femoris muscle origin. Quite a common injury in young boys. Treatment is rest.

Traumatic osteitis pubis

Traumatic osteitis pubis is a tiresome condition often seen in footballers (it is sometimes known as 'Inguinocrural pain of footballers'). The patient complains of an aching pain in the groin associated with abduction of the leg. A classic feature is marked tenderness over the symphysis pubis and the differential diagnosis is from adductor ('rider's') strain. Some cases may be associated with a genuine urethritis and may be a manifestation of Reiter's syndrome.

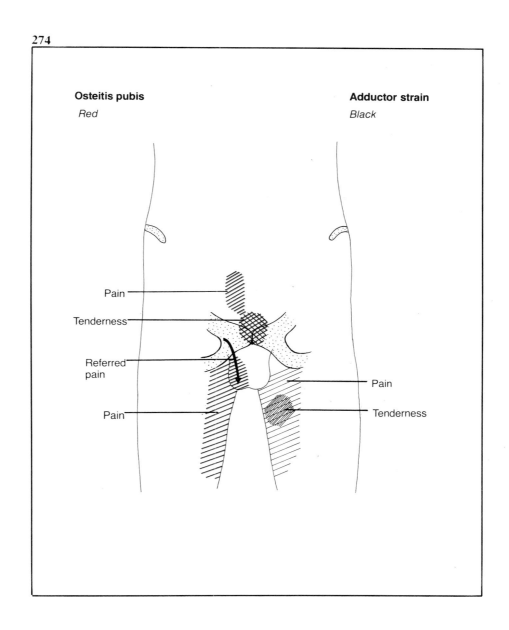

274

Osteitis pubis
Red

Adductor strain
Black

Pain

Tenderness

Referred pain

Pain

Pain

Tenderness

274 Diagramatic representation of sites of pain and tenderness (with differentiation from adductor strain).

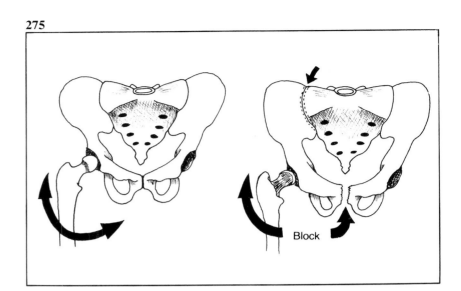

275 Mechanism of injury in extension. Inability of the distorted hip joint to rotate imposes shearing stress to the symphisis.

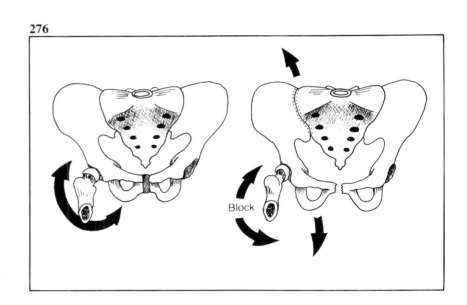

276 Mechanism of injury in flexion. In this situation the sacroiliac joints are also often involved.

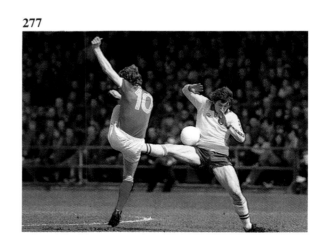

277 The stress situation. The player in red (No. 10) is at risk – the player in yellow is stressing his adductors.

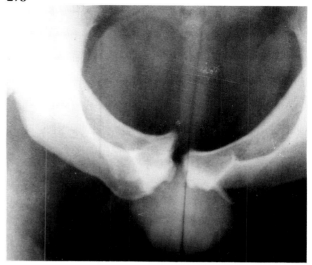

278 Traumatic osteitis pubis. Radiographic appearances of symphysis pubis.

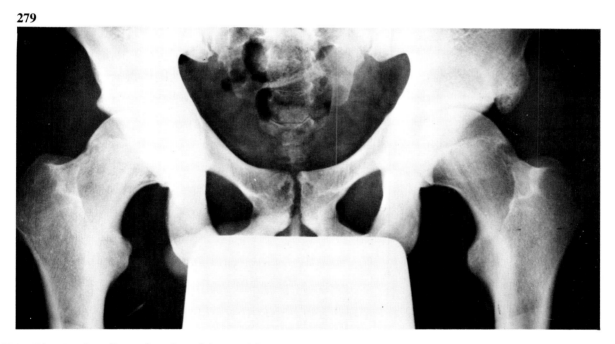

279 Pistol grip (tilt) deformity of femoral heads often associated with traumatic osteitis pubis.

Treatment is general rest, anti-inflammatory medication and hip mobilisation by exercise or manipulation.

In the really resistant case fusion of the symphysis pubis may be effective but can of itself lead to further stress due to transmission of forces onwards to the rest of the pelvis and the sacroiliac joints. Some patients show evidence, both clinical and radiological, of sacroiliac subluxation.

Ischium

Most ischial injuries in sport are like other pelvic injuries, due to avulsion of muscle attachments.

Avulsion of the hamstring is most common in the young athlete but hamstring origin strain may present at any age.

280

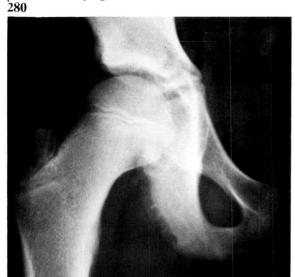

280 Hamstring tear. Radiotranslucent appearance of the ischial tuberosity associated with hamstring tear in an 11-year o^ld sprinter.

281

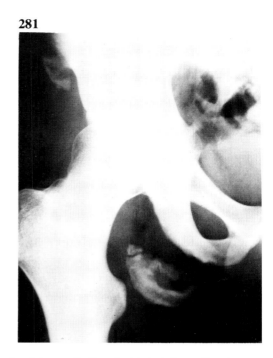

281 Avulsion of the ischial tuberosity in an adolescent schoolboy. Note also in this case avulsion of the attachment of sartorius on the same side.

282

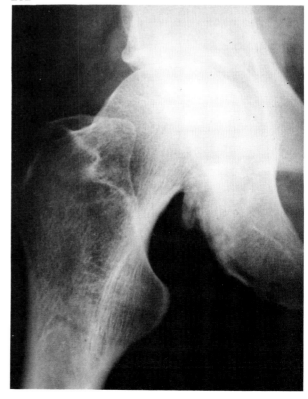

282 Calcification in the hamstring origin at the lateral end of the ischial tuberosity in a 40-year-old skier.

Muscle avulsion injuries at this site often present apparently catastrophic appearances on radiography but it is remarkable how well healing takes place with limited subsequent disability. The important aim of treatment is to stretch and mobilise the tissues within the limits of pain tolerance from the outset.

Hip joint

Degenerative joint disease

283

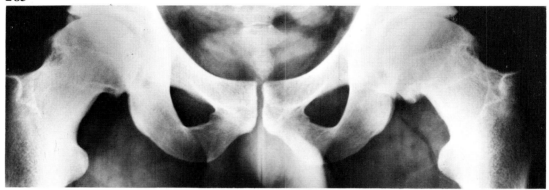

283 Severe degenerative joint disease associated with marked limitation of hip movements in an individual still playing rugby league football as a professional. Radiological appearance.

284

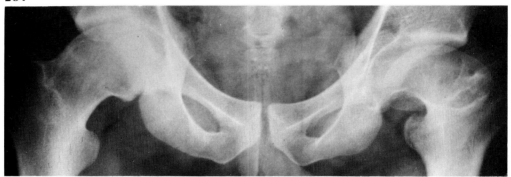

284 Dysplasia. Marked dysplasia of the hip in a professional golfer (note also deformity in other hip). Pain and discomfort in the hip during the second round of golf played in the day necessitated this individual to abandon taking part in tournament golf.

Fracture

285 Radiograph of fracture of the femur (intertrochanteric) in footballer who had fallen onto his left hip on a hard ground. He complained that the hip was sore but he was still able to walk without discomfort.

It must always be remembered that in degenerative joint disease and in other hip conditions referred pain to the knee is a presenting symptom. This is particularly important when confronted with injuries in children, when slipped upper femoral epiphysis and Perthe's disease may present.

285

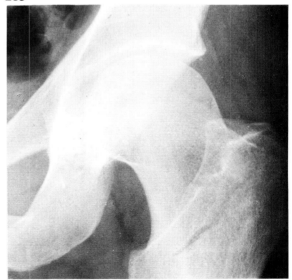

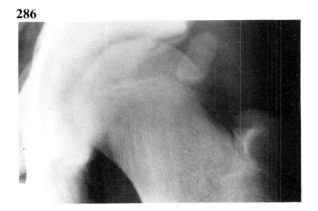

286 Fracture of the acetabular margin in a player, again a footballer, who had been tackled awkwardly and fallen across another player's leg. He continued to play football but had persistent pain.

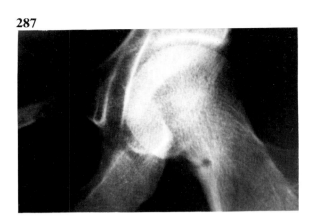

287 Stress fracture in the neck of the femur in a young badminton player.

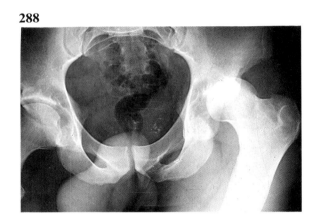

288 Dislocation of hip. Result of a fall from a horse with the foot trapped in the stirrup.

Muscle injury: adductor strain (rider's strain)

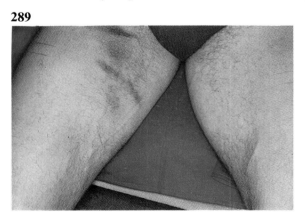

289 Ecchymosis in acute adductor strain – diffuse as in all muscle tears.

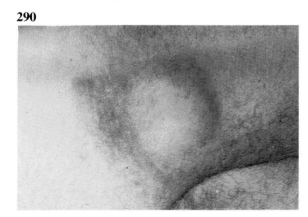

290 Ecchymosis due to direct violence (skiing) – well localised to site of blow.

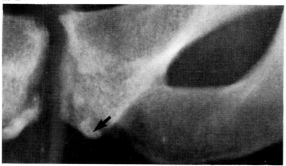

291 **Ectopic calcification** in adductor strain.

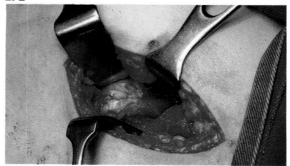

292 **Ectopic calcification** in gluteus medius tendon at operation.

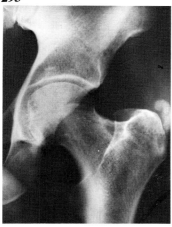

293 **Ectopic calcification** in gluteus medius tendon (trochanteric bursitis). Radiological appearance.

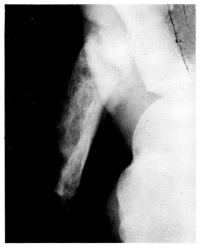

294 **Ectopic calcification** in sartorius strain – radiological appearance.

Iliotibial band syndromes

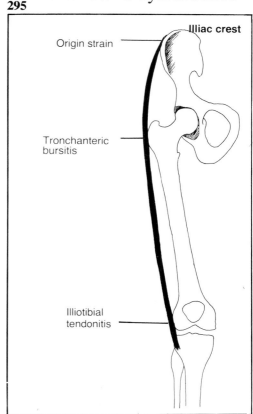

295 **Sites of injury in iliotibial band syndromes.**

Injury to the iliotibial band (tensor fascia lata) may occur as an avulsion from the origin on the iliac crest, as peritendonitis associated with trochanteric bursitis, as a muscle pull, and as a tendonitis over the lateral femoral condyle.

12   Knee joint injuries

The knee joint is the most vulnerable joint in sport being inherently unstable and fully weight-bearing. The complexity of the joint ensures a wide variety of different clinical problems. This in turn tends to produce difficulty in diagnosis, so that in some instances patients suffering from knee injury do not get the correct initial treatment and present later with degenerative joint disease.

Congenital abnormality

296

297

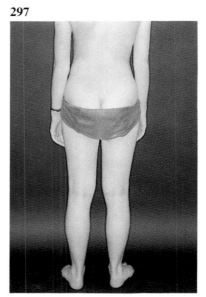

298

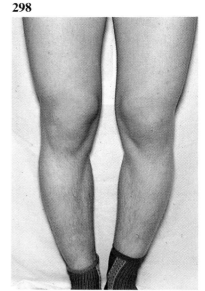

296   Genu recurvatum. Hyperextension of the knee often associated with hypermobile joint disease, and sometimes a cause of recurrent patellar dislocation.

297   Genu valgum. Knock-knee – a predisposing factor in chondromalacia patellae.

298   Genu varum. Bow-legs, often associated with torsion of the tibia.

For mechanical reasons all these abnormalities make the knee more vulnerable to trauma.

As in the case of the elbow joint varus, valgus and recurvatus deformity of the knee can impose additional mechanical stresses on the joint, in particular on the extensor apparatus which in a sportsman may lead to production of symptoms. Management may be difficult. In many instances it may be necessary to divert the patient to a more bio-mechanically suitable form of sporting activity.

Degenerative joint disease

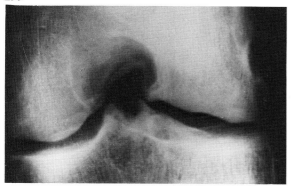

299 Osteoarthrosis associated with previous history of osteochondritis dissecans in an international weight lifter.

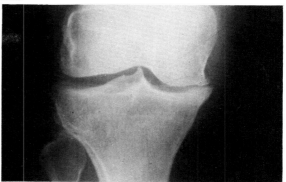

300 Osteoarthrosis of the knee joint in a 32-year-old professional tennis player who had previously had numerous injuries and a complete medial meniscectomy.

301 Osteoarthrosis of the patellofemoral joint in a footballer with long previous history of chondromalcia patellae.

Osteoarthrosis of the knee joint is relatively common at an early age in sportsmen, typically associated with inadequate or unsuitable earlier management of primary knee injury. It is therefore clearly important that all knee injuries should be taken seriously and treated and rehabilitated effectively to prevent the early onset of degenerative joint disease.

Osteochondritis dissecans

Osteochondritis dissecans is an important cause of pain in the knee in adolescent sportsmen.

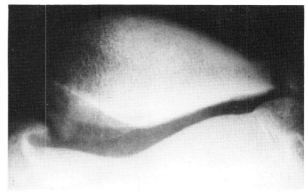

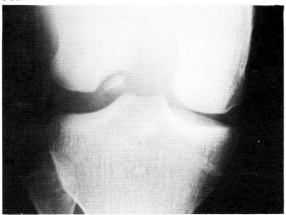

302 Condylar defect. Radiograph of knee showing marked condylar defect and loose body formation.

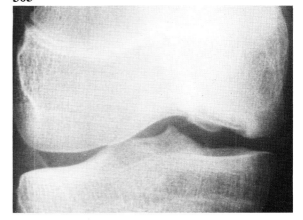

303 Fragmentation. Radiograph of knee showing less well-marked defect and early development of separating fragment. At this stage fixing the fragment may promote reattachment and subsequent healing.

304

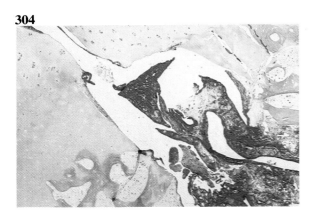

304 Histology of osteochondritic fragment.

In fact patients do surprisingly well with defects after separation (and removal) of an osteochondritic fragment. Minimal interference is the optimum line of treatment.

Knee injury – meniscus

Injury to the menisci due to rotational strain on a flexed weight-bearing knee is extremely common. Differential diagnosis and management of these injuries is according to standard orthopaedic practice.

305

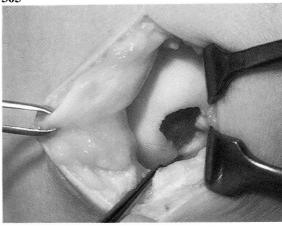

305 Erosion of femoral condyle in patient with osteochondral fracture. It is often similar in presentation and behaviour to osteochondritis dissecans – but follows acute trauma. Operative appearance.

Damage to the alar folds with nipping and tag formation may mimic meniscus tear, with apparent locking in some cases. Arthroscopy may be required to differentiate, and grossly hypertrophic alar folds may need surgical incision.

Main types of meniscus tear

306

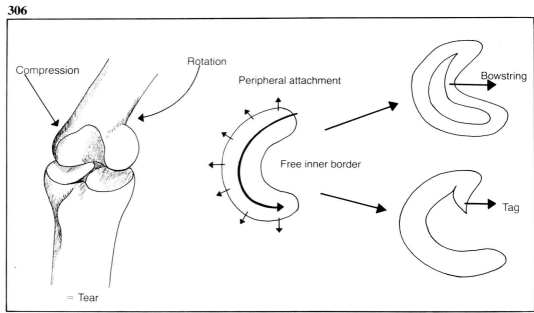

306 Mechanism of injury. Rotational stress on the flexed weight-bearing knee.

Bucket handle or 'bowstring' tear (medial meniscus).

307

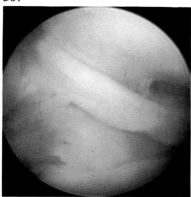

307 Tear as seen at arthroscopy.

308

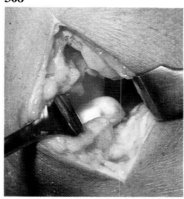

308 Tear as seen at operation for removal of detached portion.

309

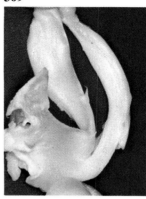

309 Menisectomy specimen showing longitudinal split. (If the periphery of the meniscus is intact it is sufficient to remove only the detached fragment.)

Tag or 'parrot beak' tear (post horn of medial meniscus).

310

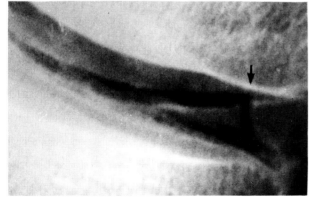

310 Tear as seen at arthrogram.

311

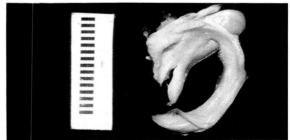

311 Tear as seen in operation specimen.

312 Chondrocalcinosis. Meniscus degeneration with ectopic calcification.

Meniscus tears are often associated with ligament damage, the effects of which are sometimes exacerbated by meniscectomy.

312

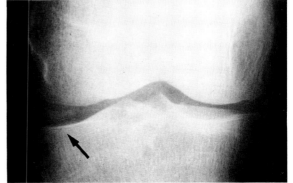

Injury to ligaments

Collateral ligament injury

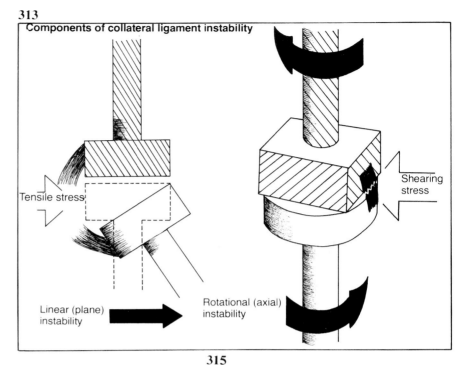

313 Components of collateral ligament instability

Tensile stress

Shearing stress

Linear (plane) instability

Rotational (axial) instability

313 Mechanism of injury. Direct stress across a ligament; may be coupled with rotational strain to give rotary instability.

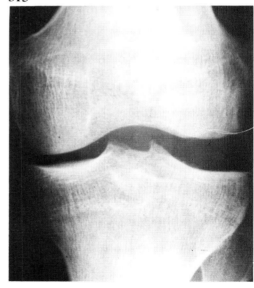

314 Medial ligament tear. Stress radiograph, showing medial side of joint opening up in medial ligament tear.

315 Lateral ligament tear. Stress radiograph, showing lateral side of joint opening up in lateral ligament tear.

Sometimes confused with lateral ligament strain is **popliteus tenosynovitis.** This condition is virtually incapable of illustration! The clinical features are pain on running downhill and on sitting with legs crossed.

Cruciate ligament injury

Cruciate ligament damage can cause severe bio-mechanical disturbance in the knee. The cruciates control not only anteroposterior movement at the knee joint but also the pivot point for rotation during the lock-home phase of extension. Damage to either cruciate, particularly when associated with capsular damage, is a potent factor of rotary instability of the knee and pivot shift. Established instability demands surgical repair. Many procedures are available for reconstruction of the anterior cruciate ligament – reconstruction of the posterior cruciate ligament in late cases is less immediately effective but alternative dynamic stabilisation procedures are available which allow resumption of normal sporting activity.

316

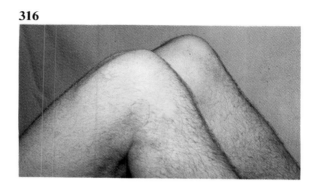

316 Posterior cruciate injury showing typical deformity of posterior drawer sign in left knee.

317

317 Anterior cruciate ligament tear. Super-imposed lateral radiograph showing instability in cruciate ligament tear.

318   **319**   **320**

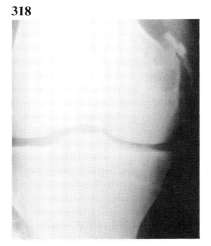 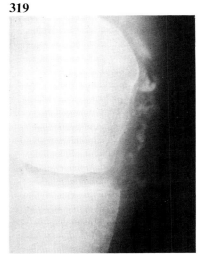 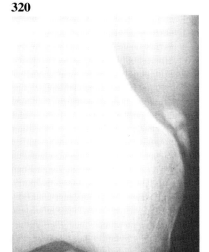

318 Ectopic calcification in the upper attachment of the medial collateral ligament.

Ectopic calcification in the upper attachment of the medial collateral ligament is sometimes a sequel of injury. The radiological appearances are variable.

319 Pellegrini – Stieda's disease: a variant.

320 Pellegrini – Stieda's disease: a further variant.

In all cases calcification is present. When symptomatic, local steroid injection usually cures.

Coronary ligament stain. Occasionally the coronary ligaments binding the menisci to the upper surface of the tibia may be strained. Symptoms are similar to meniscus tear, but without locking, and tenderness is below the joint line. Treatment is conservative.

Reconstruction of ligaments after knee injury

Effective reconstruction after severe ligament damage to the knee joint with instability demands a clear understanding of the nature of the damage and the mechanical instability produced. Provided effective diagnosis of the nature of the instability is achieved, restoration of function will follow appropriate reconstruction using established orthopaedic techniques.

Patients with both functional and clinical instability of the knee as a result of ligament injury almost invariably require surgical stabilisation for their return to normal sporting activity. Many procedures are available to meet the wide range of different combinations of ligament damage, and each has its own protagonist. Knee reconstructions fall into two basic types – static and dynamic.

In static reconstruction the object of treatment is to reconstruct the ligament, either directly by repair or by replacement using autogenous or other materials. By contrast, dynamic repair involves the realignment of a muscle so that by altering its action, a stabilising force may be applied to the joint in the appropriate direction.

Examples of operation for stabilisation

The pes anserinus transfer is a classic example of stabilisation based on modified muscle function. In this instance the knee flexors of the pes anserinus by their re-insertion become medial rotators of the knee and on extension, the conjoint tendon of the pes anserinus stabilises the medial collateral ligament.

It must be remembered that ligamentous instability is often compound and in the case of anteromedial rotary instability pes anserinus transfer may be inadequate by itself. The patient may require some form of medial capsular plication or medial ligament reconstruction (as has been carried out in **332**). Some form of reinforcement of the posteromedial capsule of the knee may also be required as in the 'five-in-one' procedure.

321 and 322   Dynamic: Pes anserinus transfer for medial rotary instability (operation and diagram). Stability of knee is maintained by active muscular contraction.

321

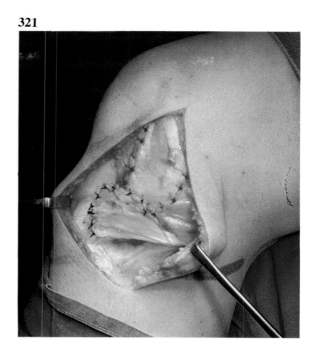

322

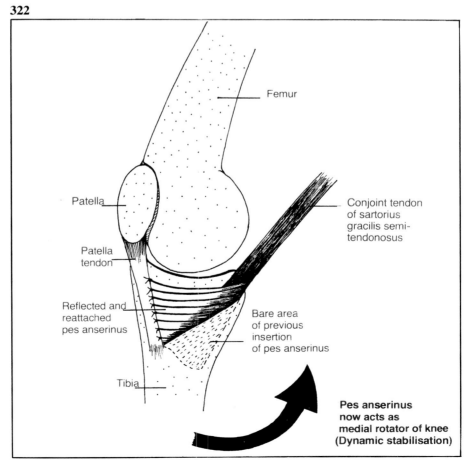

97

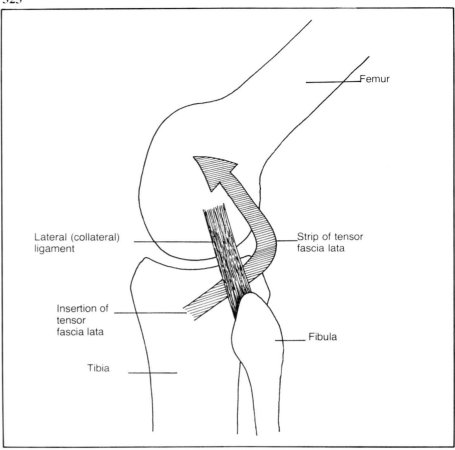

323 Static stabilisation McIntosh repair for lateral rotary instability (diagram and operation). Stability of the knee maintained by reconstructed ligament.

Femur

Lateral (collateral) ligament

Strip of tensor fascia lata

Insertion of tensor fascia lata

Fibula

Tibia

323 Static stabilisation McIntosh repair for lateral rotary instability (diagram and operation). Stability of the knee maintained by reconstructed ligament.

After reconstruction a carefully graded rehabilitation programme is essential to rebuild muscle and re-educate proprioceptive feedback.

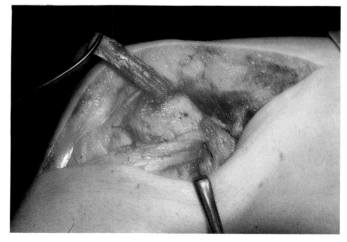

324

324 McIntosh procedure. Essentially a strip of tensor fascia lata is passed backwards deep to the lateral collateral ligament to pull the lateral condyle backwards – a static stabilisation.

Swellings of the knee joint

Swellings outside the knee joint are quite common and may cause confusion.

325

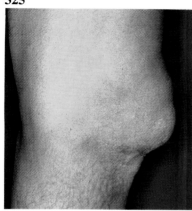

326

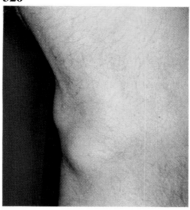

327

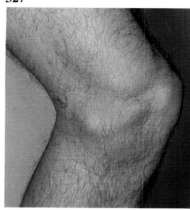

325 Pre-patellar bursitis (housemaid's knee). Often traumatic and may develop as a result of an abrasion on hard ground or a wrestling mat.

326 Popliteal cyst. So called 'Baker's cyst' or gastrocnemius bursa. The cyst may arise as a pouch from the posterior capsule of the knee (with which it may communicate) or it may be associated with the semi-membranosus tendon or gastrocnemius. Differential diagnosis is from popliteal aneurysm which pulsates.

327 Cystic meniscus. This condition is commonly found on the lateral side. Occasionally it occurs on the medial side.

328

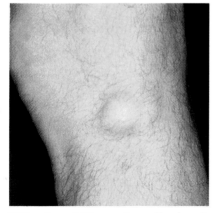

329

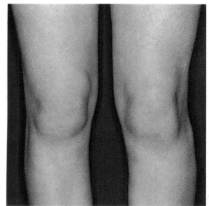

328 An oddity – a 'ganglion' or bursa associated with the superior tibio-fibular joint which could be mistaken for a cyst of lateral meniscus.

329 Sesamoid. A solid one. A prominent fibular head with an accessory ossicle (sesamoid) in the biceps tendon.

These conditions are essentially benign and need no treatment other than reassurance, except if there is interference with mechanical function or pain due to tension in a cyst. In such instances surgical removal may be required.

Aspiration of cystic swellings is *not* recommended except as a 'one off' emergency procedure, due to the liability to cause loculation.

13 Patella injuries

Chondromalacia

Chondromalacia patellae is very common in sportsmen. Males are more commonly affected than females (a reversal of the ratio in the normal population). The condition is typically associated with impaired function of the extensor apparatus of the knee and is relatively easily treated provided that its biomechanical basis is understood.

Chondromalacia may be quite protean in its presentation and may mimic a variety of other conditions including meniscus tear. It is also commonly present in association with other conditions such as meniscus tear, chronic traumatic synovitis, etc.

330

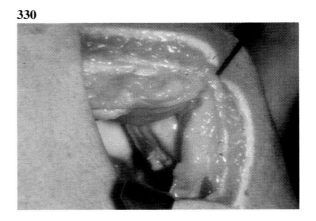

330 Patella. Under-surface of the patella at arthrotomy showing typical degenerative change. The changes on the undersurface of the patella are to be regarded merely as an indicator of altered patellofemoral biomechanics. They are of no significance in symptom production. Attempts to treat chondromalacia patellae by direct intervention on the undersurface of the patella are therefore unrewarding.

331

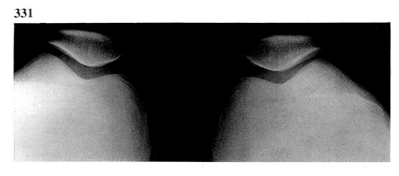

331 Patella. Skyline radiograph showing typical lateral tilt or sub-luxation of patella associated with chondromalacia patellae.

332

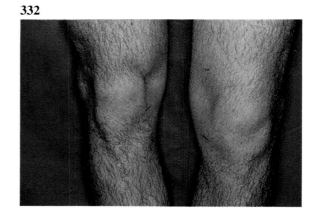

332 Vastus medialis wasting. A cardinal feature of chondromalacia patellae. Vastus medialis wasting is of itself a product of inability fully to extend the knee which is in turn a consequence of any form of irritation of the knee joint, slight effusion or synovitis. The vicious circle of symptom production in chondromalacia with vastus medialis wasting and loss of normal patellofemoral joint congruity is clearly readily established as a result of even minor knee injuries.

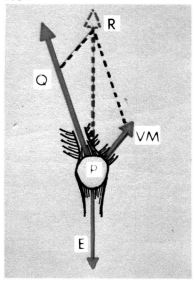

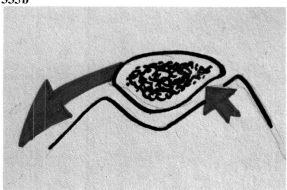

333 Biomechanics of extension. (a) The angle QPR is the Q angle. Note that with the knee extended the pull of the vastus medialis (VM) counteracts the tendency of the patella to displace laterally in extension; the result of the forces of the pull on the quadriceps tendon and the vastus medialis lies in the axis of patella tendon (E). (b) Stabilisation of patella is partly passive by the lateral condylar ridge.

334

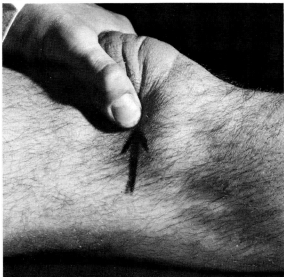

335

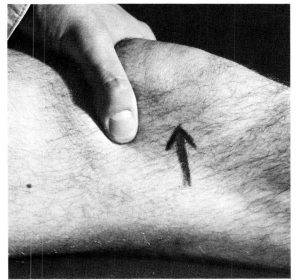

334 and 335 Eliciting Clarke's sign. The leg is fully extended and the patient is told to relax. The patella is then pressed downwards and distally onto the patella femoral groove. The patient experiences pain when the quadriceps is now contracted. This sign is pathognomonic of chondromalacia patellae. Note the patient should be warned to contract the quadriceps *gently*.

Apart from trauma causing quadriceps inhibition, predisposing factors include the following:

336

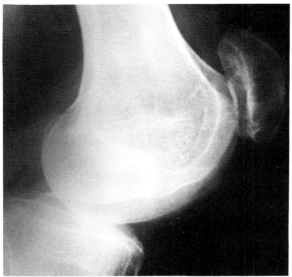

337

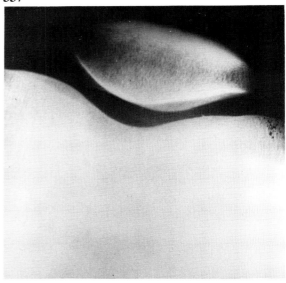

336 Patella alta (long patella tendon). The patella rides so high it loses the passive stabilisation by the lateral condylar ridge.

337 Small patella (often with recurrent dislocation). Note small patella not engaging properly on the (in this case shallow) femoral articular surface.

338

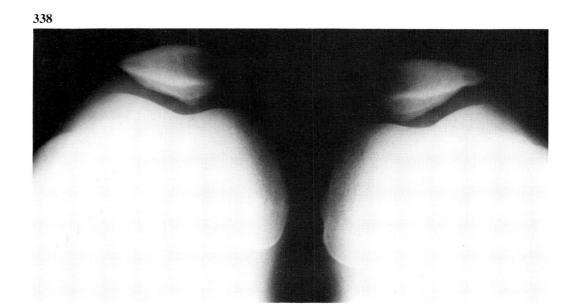

338 Abnormal shape (e.g. Wiberg type III with virtually no medial condylar facet). The pull of the quadriceps tends to 'squint' the patella laterally.

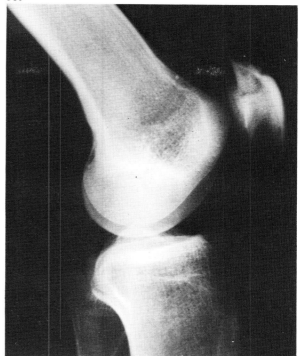

339 Bipartite patella. The accessory fragment is notoriously prone to malacic changes (see **346**).

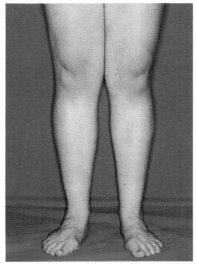

340 Genu valgum. The increased valgus angle in extension (Q angle) multiplies the resultant tendency to displace the patella laterally (parallelogram of forces).

The presence of any of these conditions will materially affect the biomechanics of the extensor apparatus, tending to increase the Q angle and facilitate subluxation of the patella.

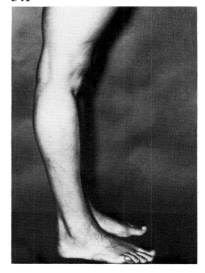

341 Genu recurvatum. The patella loses its seating on the lower end of the femur in hyper-extension.

Conservative management

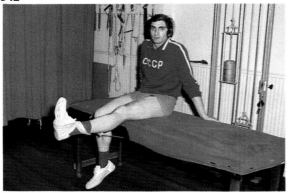

342   Vigorous static quadriceps contraction restores vastus medialis. Since vastus medialis only effectively functions in full or nearly full extension, it can only effectively be exercised with the knee extended.

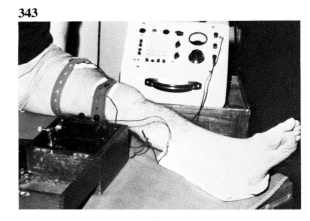

343   Vastus medialis. Occasionally this muscle is severely inhibited; feedback may be secured by Faradic stimulation including sequential faradism in which the vastus medialis is stimulated slightly in advance of the main mass of the quadriceps.

Surgical management

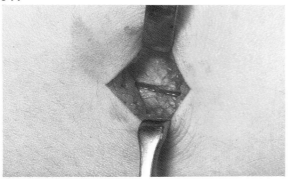

344   Lateral retinacular release. This is the simplest procedure. It may be carried out through a small incision on the lateral side of the knee or through an arthroscopy incision; the capsulotomy.

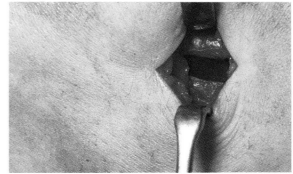

345   The capsulotomy completed. Note gap as a result of medial shift of the patella.

Other biomechanically sound procedures, such as anterior tibial transposition, may be helpful. Procedures such as drilling the bone, patellar shave and even patellectomy are not biomechanically sound and results are frequently poor.

Chondromalacia patellae is one of the commonest complaints in sport and represents up to 10 per cent of all problems seen in sports injuries clinics. It is relatively easy to treat provided its biomechanical cause is understood, but it is yet remarkable how commonly the condition is inadequately managed and patients persist with symptoms. The condition is most notorious when it presents in adolescent and late-teenage girls, particularly those who are somewhat endomorphic and have a tendency to genu valgum. Too often these patients come finally to patellectomy as a result of inadequate early management and the results are monotonously disappointing. In the early cases shortwave diathermy together with appropriate muscle re-education will normally produce the required relief of symptoms. Lateral Retinacular Release should be regarded as the primary surgical treatment of choice in the patient who fails to respond to conservative management.

Patella-bipartite

This development anomaly is sometimes confused with a fracture. It typically involves the upper outer pole of the patella. The articular surface of the fragment is often malacic and associated with recalcitrant symptoms.

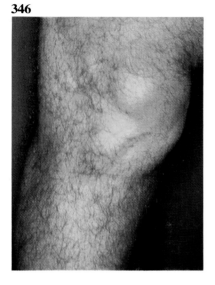

346 Patella. Clinical appearance showing visible and palpable boss on superolateral aspect of patella.

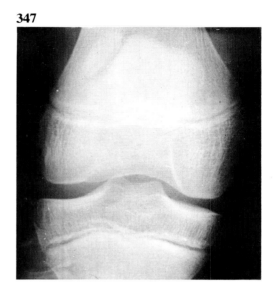

347 Patella. Anteroposterior view. Radiographic appearance. Not to be confused with a fracture!

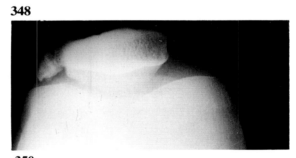

348 Patella. Skyline radiograph showing displacement of accessory fragment.

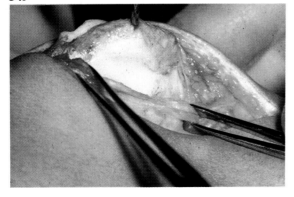

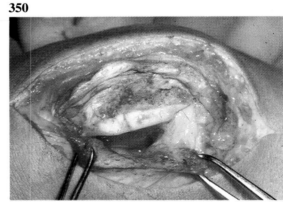

349 and 350 Appearance at operation for removal of the fragment. Most cases are untroubled by symptoms. When they occur the patient should be managed as for chondromalacia patellae. Excision of the fragment combined with lateral retinacular release is valuable in recalcitrant cases.

Osteochondritis

Osteochondritis of the patella is relatively uncommon but it is seen as a form of traction epiphysitis (Sinding–Larsen–Johanssen syndrome) and also as osteochondritis dissecans affecting the articular surface.

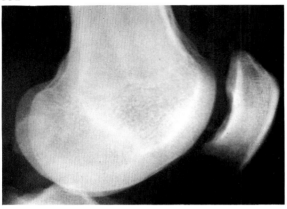

351

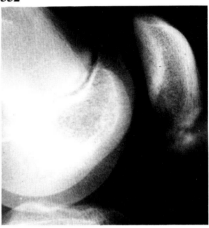

352

351 Osteochondritis dissecans. Lateral radiograph showing defect on the posterior surface of the patella and a loose body visible in the posterior compartment of the knee between the femoral condyles. Treatment is excision of the loose body. The defect in the patella can usually be left alone.

352 Sinding–Larsen–Johannsen disease showing typical appearances of osteochondritis at the lower pole of the patella. This is a condition often associated with overuse, the treatment for which is rest. It is the juvenile equivalent of jumper's knee (**361**).

Fracture of the patella

353

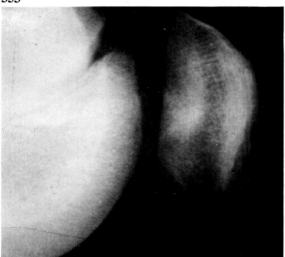

354

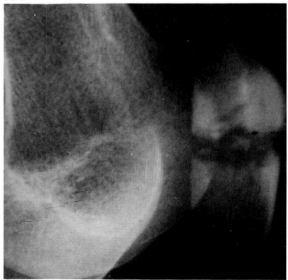

353 Stress fracture of the lower pole of the patella showing avulsion of the superficial cortex.

354 Fracture of the patella. Shown on lateral radiograph through the middle of the patella. This is due to indirect violence, i.e. the pull of the quadriceps apparatus. This patient returned to international football after excision of the distal fragment and reconstruction of the capsule and extensor apparatus.

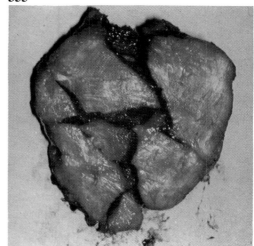

355 Fracture of the patella. Comminuted fracture due to direct violence. Attempts at reduction and realignment of fragments with or without fixation are seldom as fruitful as patellectomy. The latter will, however, usually effectively preclude further body-contact sport.

Dislocation of the patella

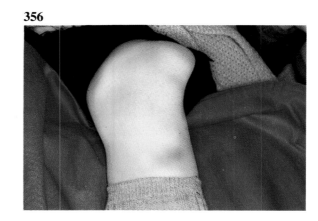

356 Clinical appearance. Note obvious deformity. The dislocation is usually easy to reduce as long as the knee can be extended.

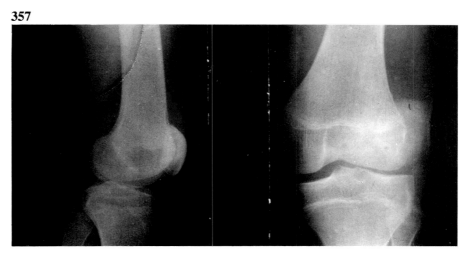

357 Radiographical appearance. A similar confusing appearance may be suggested in anteroposterior radiographs of the knee which are not well centred.

Predisposing factors in patellar dislocation are, not surprisingly, the same as those for chondromalacia patellae (**336** to **341**).

Patella Tendon

Patella tendonitis – jumper's knee

Patellar tendonitis is common in sports involving much jumping, and is characterised by pain and tenderness below the knee cap and over the patella tendon.

358 a, b and c Examples of sports involving jumping a) volley ball; b) basket ball; c) athletics.

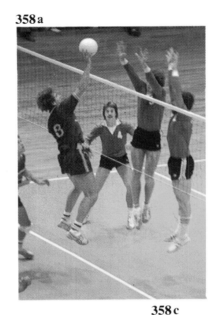

358 a

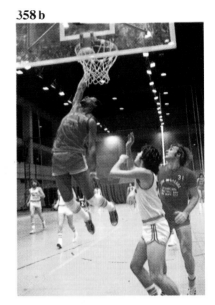

358 b

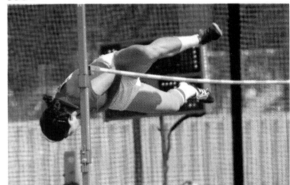

358 c

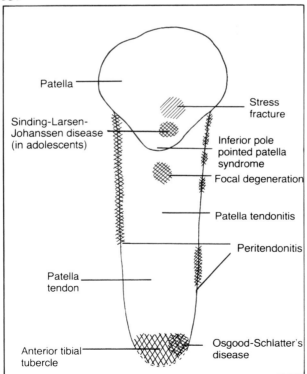

359 Differential diagnosis of patellar tendon pain.

Patella

Sinding-Larsen-Johanssen disease (in adolescents)

Patella tendon

Anterior tibial tubercle

Stress fracture

Inferior pole pointed patella syndrome

Focal degeneration

Patella tendonitis

Peritendonitis

Osgood-Schlatter's disease

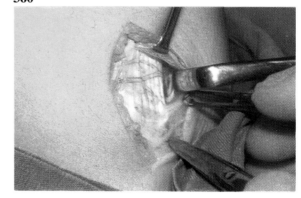

360 Peritendonitis of the patella tendon. Note adhesions between tendon and surrounding tissues.

361

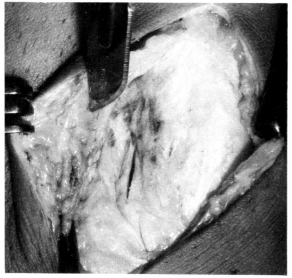

361 Tendonitis of the patella tendon. The tendon is diffusely thickened and tender.

362

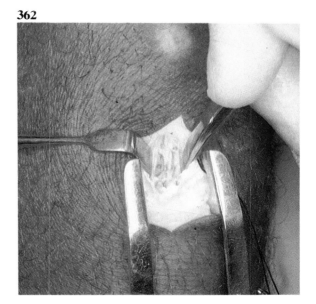

362 Focal degeneration of the patella tendon. A lesion demonstrated at operation (decathlete).

363

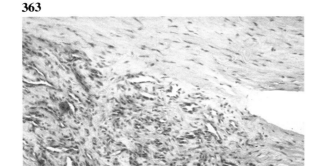

363 Histology of patella tendon focal degeneration. Note typical 'wet tissue paper' appearance with increased cells and new blood vessel formation.

364

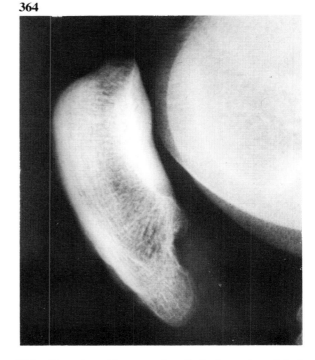

364 Prominent lower pole – 'inferior pole pointed syndrome'. Radiological appearance. Clinically similar to 'jumper's knee', it presents with tenderness at lower pole of patella.

These conditions may respond to conservative treatment, e.g. anti-inflammatory medication, ultrasonics or shortwave diathermy. Recalcitrant cases require surgical exploration. Chondromalacia patellae is a frequent complication.

Patella tendon insertion

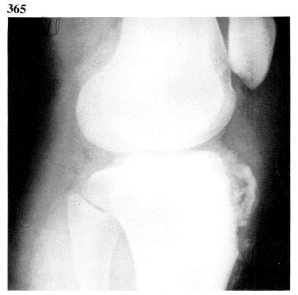

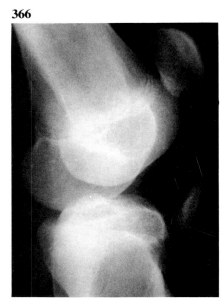

365 Osgood-Schlatter's disease, possibly due to excessive tension in the patella tendon insertion on the epiphysis of the anterior tibial tubercle in adolescence as a result of overtraining. Note fragmentation of epiphysis. In some cases these separated fragments may have to be surgically removed to secure relief of pain.

Old Osgood–Schlatter's disease. Abnormally prominent anterior tibial tubercle.

366 Avulsion of the anterior tibial tubercle. The consequence of acute overloading.

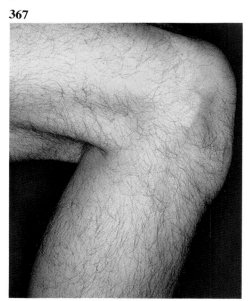

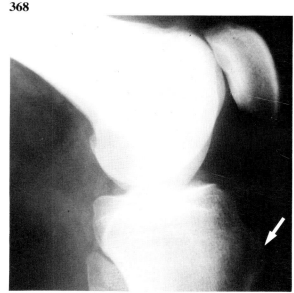

367 Clinical appearance.

368 Radiological appearance.

Usually of no significance but may be vulnerable to knocks and kicks.

14 Lower leg injuries

Lower limb injuries in sport are extremely common, both as a result of direct and indirect violence and of overuse. Apart from basic fractures and soft-tissue injuries, a number of special conditions are met in sport which may cause problems.

Differential diagnosis is sometimes difficult unless the particular mechanism of the sport involved is borne in mind. It is important to note that a number of painful conditions in the lower limb may be associated with foot deformities. This is particularly true of the inflammatory lesions affecting the stirrup tendons and the muscles that power them.

Stress fractures

369

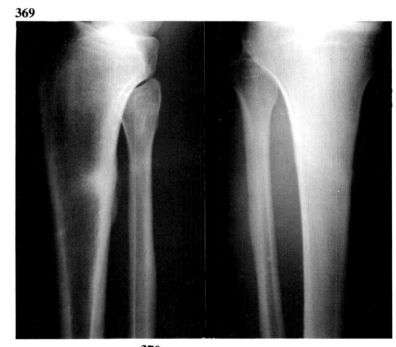

369 Typical appearance of stress fracture in the junction of the upper and middle thirds of the tibia in a 400-metre track athlete.

370

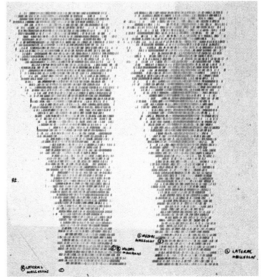

370 Technetium 99 bone scan showing 'hot node' in tibia.

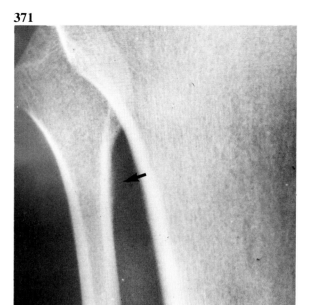

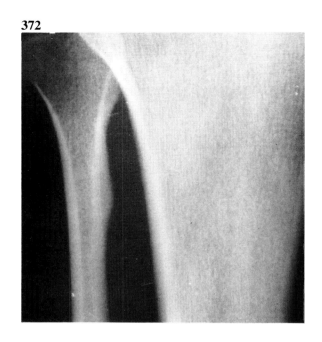

371 and 372   Development of fibula stress fracture. Radiological appearances at dates 9.77 (three weeks after onset of symptoms) and 4.78.

373

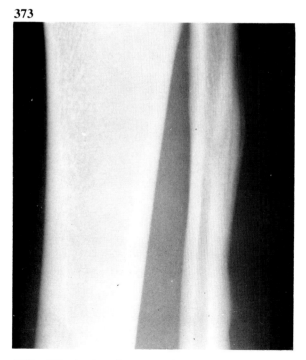

374

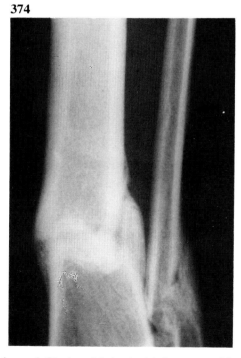

373   Fibula showing stress fracture at the junction of middle and lower thirds in a footballer.

Management of stress fractures always involves reduction of cessation of stressful activity as well as symptomatic measures.

374   Tibia and fibula. United old fracture with recent stress fracture visible in the fibula above the site of the original fracture. Stress fracture in the fibula is a not uncommon problem in patients undergoing intensive rehabilitation for return to sport after major fractures of the lower limb.

375 Anterior tibial cortical hyperplasia. The other stress response, usually painful and difficult to differentiate from stress fracture. Note marked narrowing of medullary canal: a marathon runner. This condition can be a source of considerable disability particularly in middle-distance and long-distance runners. Apart from reducing the mileage little can be done by way of conservative management. However, recent studies suggest that drilling of the thickened cortical bone (2.5mm drill holes at a separation of 2cm) produces a remarkable relief of symptoms and early resumption of training within a matter of a few weeks.

375

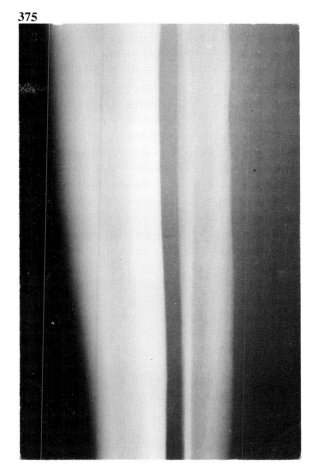

376

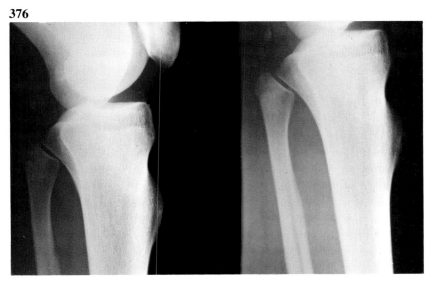

376 Benign exostosis. *Not* Osgood–Schlatter's. A benign exostosis vulnerable to knocks playing football.

Shin pain

Shin pain, otherwise known as 'shin splints' or 'shin soreness' is a portmanteau term referring to the symptom of pain in the anterior aspect of the lower leg. The conditions involved are essentially due to overuse and may be acute, as in the case of anterior tibial compartment syndrome, but are more commonly chronic.

377

Stress fracture localised

Posterior tibial syndrome (levels usually afflicted)

Tibia

Anterior tibial compartment syndrome

Anterior tibial cortical hyperplasia (diffuse)

Stress fracture

Anterior tibial tenosynovitis

Extensor retinaculum entrapment syndrome

Posterior tibial tendovaginitis

377   Differential diagnosis of shin pain.

Posterior tibial syndrome

Posterior tibial syndrome (sometimes known as medial tibial syndrome) due to tearing away of the muscle fascia from the medial border of the tibia, with subsequent scar tissue formation.

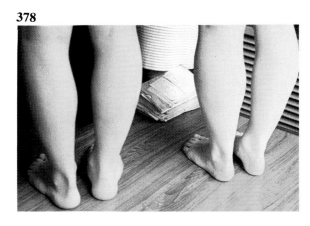

378   Posterior tibial syndrome. This type of leg with the low soleus insertion is typical of the patient with posterior tibial syndrome.

Decompression of the posterior tibial compartment relieves pain, permitting free movement of the muscles within. Similar types of procedure can be used for anterior tibial compartment syndrome.

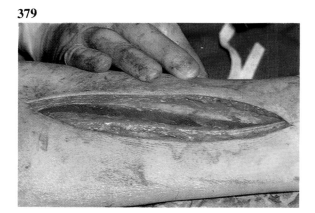

379   Extensive open decompression for posterior tibial compartment syndrome. The patient has subsequently competed as a cross-country running international.

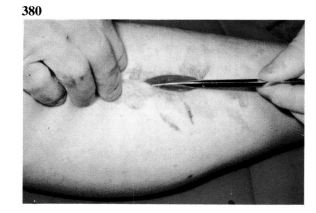

380 Closed decompression using a special fasciotome which leaves a smaller neater scar.

Diverse problems

Other problems involving the lower leg from time to time cause a degree of diagnostic confusion. The most important thing to remember is that there is a wide variety of possibilities and that many cases of pain are associated with disorders of gait, often due to constitutional structural anomalies in the leg or foot.

381

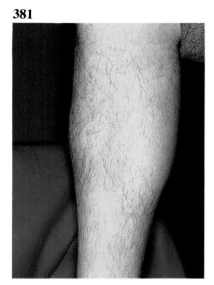

381 Subperiosteal haematoma as a result of a direct blow on the front of the shin. A hockey player.

382

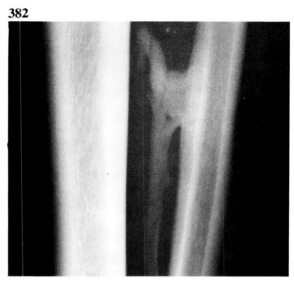

382 Ectopic calcification. Radiograph. Cause unknown in this middle-distance runner. The patient complained of persistent pain and inability to train.

383

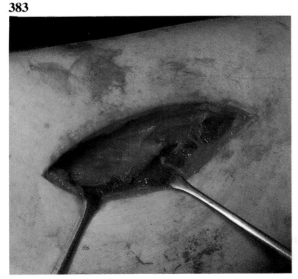

383 Cock's-comb tibia. Operation photograph showing removal of 'cock's-comb' exostosis of tibia also associated with pain on running. The patient subsequently resumed his sport pain free.

384

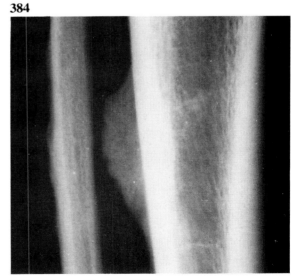

384 Xray of lesion (383).

385

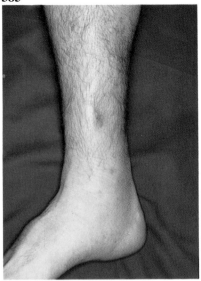

385 Localised haematoma. Small localised haematomata are very common over the shin and are often associated with the failure of absorption of the extravasated blood, leading to the development of cysts filled with dark 'blackcurrant jelly' clots. These haematomata disolve very slowly if managed conservatively, so the treatment of choice is surgical evacuation.

387

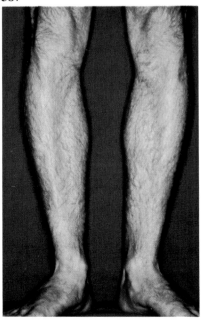

387 Tibial torsion. This patient was convinced he was a born marathon runner! Another example of tibial torsion associated with valgus feet.

386

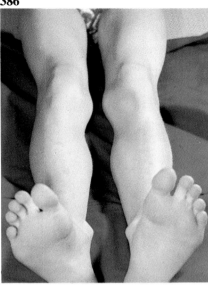

386 Tibial torsion. Note 'squinting patallae' in young swimmer with pain during dolphin kick in butterfly stroke.

388

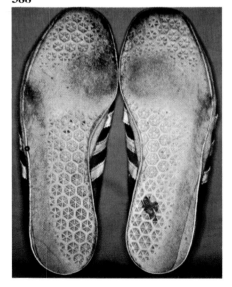

388 Uneven wear on the shoes of a patient with valgus feet (**387**). Normal wear is from outer side of heel to inner side of sole.

15 Achilles tendon injuries

Achilles tendon pain is a problem in sport. Complete rupture is usually intrinsic but the patient often complains that he has been struck on the back of the leg. The diagnosis should be clearcut except in the untreated chronic case, where blood-clot bridging the gap between the tendon ends may cast some doubts. The main problem is in differentiating between lesions of the tendon and those of the surrounding tissues (paratenon). Differentiation is usually relatively easy with the movement test. Many of the pathological changes in Achilles tendon pain can co-exist – for example, focal degeneration and chronic peritendonitis.

The movement test

389

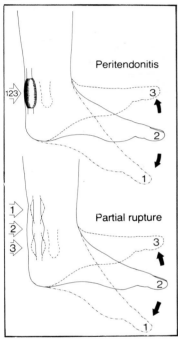

389 Differential diagnosis of tendon and paratenon lesions. Diagrammatic representation of the fixed position of the swelling and inflammation of peritendonitis as compared with the obvious movement of the lesion within the tendon with excursion of the foot.

390

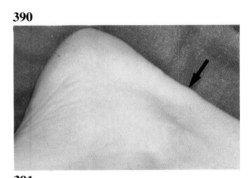

391

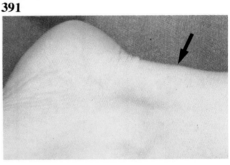

390 and 391 A tendon lesion with foot in neutral and full plantar flexion. Note obvious movement of point of swelling in the tendon in relation to the medial malleolus.

Complete rupture

392

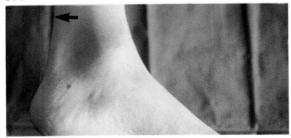

392 Ruptured tendon. Clinical appearance. Note obvious 'dent' in tendon outline proximal to stump of tendon (arrowed).

Although conservative management has its protagonists, the optimum treatment for complete

393

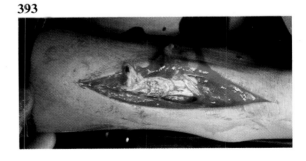

393 Tendon damage as demonstrated at operation for surgical repair.

rupture in sportsmen is almost invariably surgical repair.

Partial rupture

394

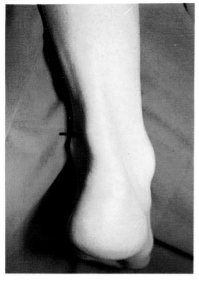

395

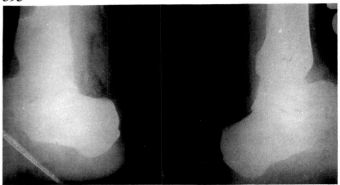

395 X-ray showing distortion of soft-tissue shadow and some infiltration of Karger's triangle. The latter is a sign of reaction in the tissues surrounding the tendon.

394 The clinical appearances are similar to tendonitis, but will depend upon the extent of the damage.

Different types of partial rupture

396 Minor partial rupture on the subcutaneous surface. A jogger.

396

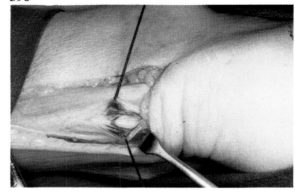

397

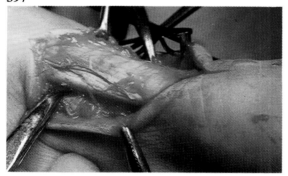

398

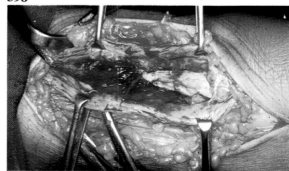

397 Partial rupture extending into the tendon but with no gross loss of continuity. An international footballer.

398 Gross partial rupture with loss of continuity of the gastrocnemius components. A netball player.

Partial rupture is always of sudden onset. The treatment depends on the extent of the rupture and the disability it causes. In minor cases it may be

managed as focal degeneration (see below), but a period of immobilisation in plaster-of-Paris (with surgery in severe cases) is often required.

Focal degeneration

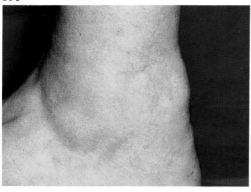

399 Focal degeneration. Clinical appearance. Note well·localised swelling on tendon.

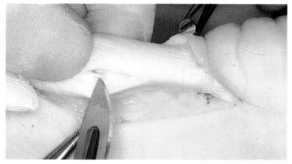

401 Operative photograph showing small area of degeneration with granulation tissue in the centre of the tendon. A 400-metres runner.

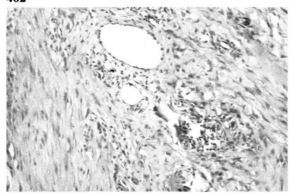

402 Histological appearance. Note 'wet tissue paper effect' with lacunae in the tendon tissue and new blood vessel formation.

Symptoms of focal degeneration develop insidiously. The condition appears to be the result of repeated microtrauma (overuse injury) in a

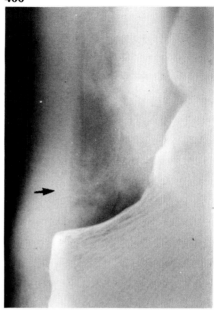

400 Focal degeneration. Radiological appearance. The soft-tissue shadow of the tendon shows a fusiform expansion.

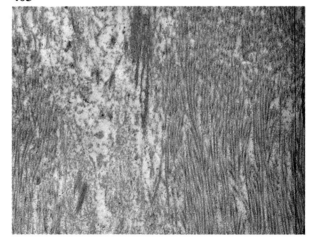

403 Electron microscopy showing organelles associated with tissue damage and darker threads of disordered elastin. Note normal collagen banding.

relatively avascular tissue which does not allow for adequate or effective healing. In established cases tenolysis is required.

Tendonitis

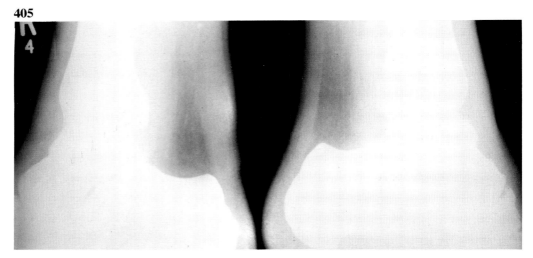

404 Achilles tendonitis. Clinical photograph showing typical diffuse swelling; palpable subcutaneously.

405 Radiographic appearance showing thickening of the soft-tissue shadow of the tendon but no infiltration of Karger's triangle.

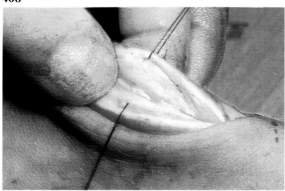

406 Appearance at operation. Without tourniquet showing loss of normal glistening appearance and bulging of cut surfaces due to local oedema. A jogger.

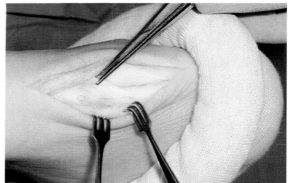

407 Operation under tourniquet showing discoloration due to haemorrhage into the tendon. A footballer.

Onset of symptoms in tendonitis is also gradual. The tendon is more widely and diffusely tender and swollen. This will more readily respond to rest, a heel raise and physiotherapy.

Peritendonitis

408

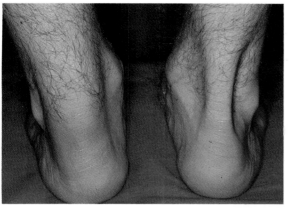

408 Diffuse thickening around the Achilles tendon typical of Achilles peritendonitis.

409

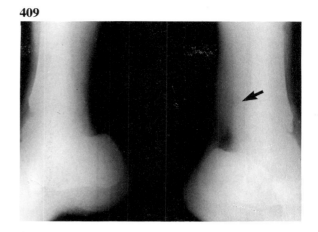

409 Soft-tissue radiograph of the Achilles tendon showing obliteration of Karger's triangle.

Peritendonitis when acute (often with crepitus) usually responds well to multipoint injections of local anaesthetic and hyaluronidase. Steroids are seldom needed!

When chronic and fibrotic, surgery becomes virtually the only means of securing return to full activity.

Note that in some cases the adherent chronically scarred paratenon may become so grossly thickened as not only to cause irritation due to friction between tendon and paratenon but so as mechanically to limit excursion of the tendon within the sheath. Excision of the paratenon does not appear significantly to prejudice the blood supply of the tendon in these cases.

410

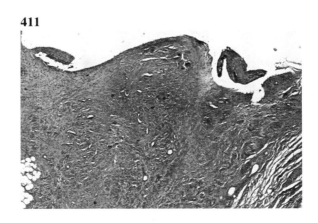

410 Operative view showing dense adhesions round Achilles tendon. A 1500 metres international runner.

411

411 Histology of paratenon showing evidence of old and new scar-tissue formation, deposits of fibrin, and extravasated blood.

Bursitis

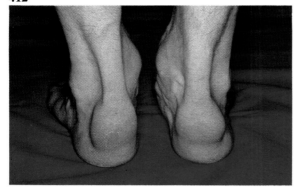

412 **Typical clinical appearance** of Achilles tendon bursitis, often associated with ill-fitting sports shoes.

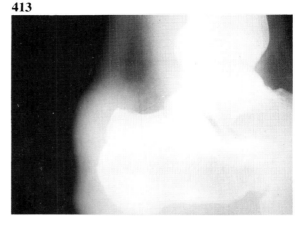

413 **Radiological appearance** of Achilles tendon bursitis showing swelling marked by soft-tissue shadow.

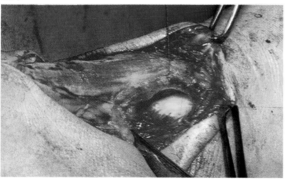

414 **Operative appearance of bursa** deep to the Achilles tendon. This is associated with a mass of granulation tissue within the bursa that requires curettage.

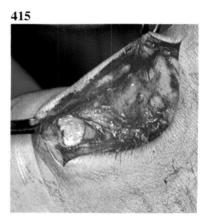

415 **Operative appearance of Achilles bursa** superficial to the tendon. The bursa has been packed with gauze to demonstrate its cavity more readily.

Calcified bursitis

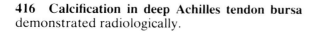

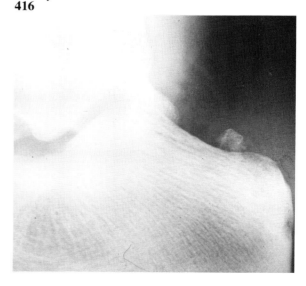

416 **Calcification in deep Achilles tendon bursa** demonstrated radiologically.

Early cases will respond to shortwave diathermy. When chronic, surgical excision may be necessary. In all cases attention must be paid to the need for suitable footwear.

Insertion lesions

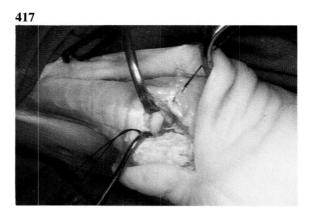

417 Insertion lesion. Operative photograph showing nidus of granulation tissue in erosion of the Achilles tendon insertion. Probably a chronic traction injury.

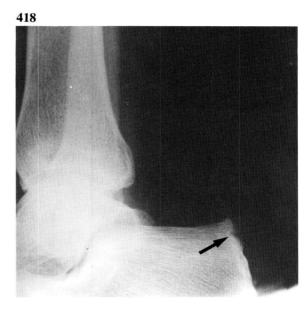

418 Radiograph showing small erosion in the posterior aspect of the calcaneum associated with Achilles insertion lesion. Resistant cases may require surgical curettage.

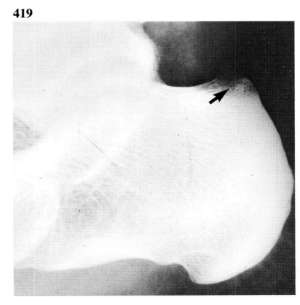

419 Radiograph of heel showing small exostosis at the Achilles tendon insertion, often associated with chronic deep Achilles tendon bursa.

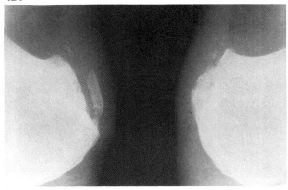

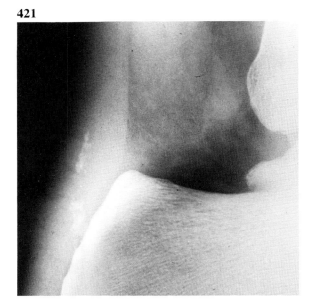

420 **Ectopic calcification** in the Achilles tendon at its insertion.

421 **Ectopic calcification** in tendon itself. Radiological appearance. In some instances actual bone may be laid down.

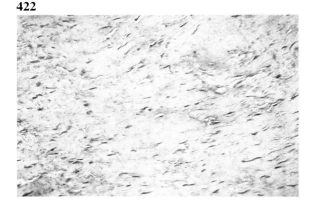

422 **Ectopic chondrification** in tendon. Histology showing cartilage deposit in degenerate Achilles tendon.

Musculotendonous junction

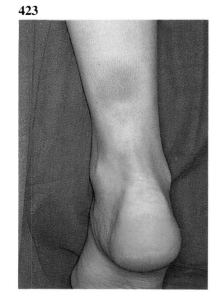

Partial tears of the musculotendonous junction (as indeed tears in the gastrocnemius more proximally) are often misdiagnosed as 'ruptured plantaris tendon'. The latter condition has not in fact been shown to exist. Treatment of musculotendonous junction injury is in accordance with the usual management of muscle or tendon injury, depending on the component structure most affected.

423 **Clinical appearance of musculotendonous junction** lesion showing bruising of overlying skin: a long jumper. This lesion is an acute instantaneous intrinsic injury very similar to a muscle tear and the result of unco-ordinated explosive effort.

Scar problems

Achilles tendon surgery has become more popular in efforts to restore function to sportsmen suffering from chronic Achilles tendon pain. It is not without its problems, most of which relate to the skin wound. This is an area notorious for poor healing.

Wound dehiscence may occur with too energetic mobilisation in the early stages, particularly if the patient tries to do too much on his own. The chronic problem is hypertrophic scar-tissue formation.

424

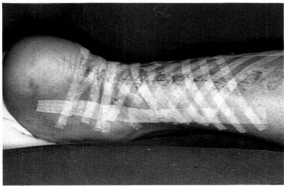

424 Immediate postoperative photograph showing wound closed with 'Steristrips'. These are used to distribute the strain over the surrounding skin and to avoid the use of sutures, which are liable to cause wound necrosis.

425

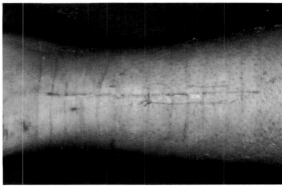

425 Clinical photograph immediately after removal of 'Steristrips' on 12th postoperative day.

426

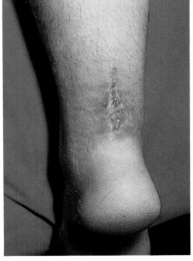

426 Early postoperative complication. Wound dehiscence (typically at the lower end) often associated with uncontrolled and excessive activity during the early postoperative (two to three weeks) rehabilitation phase. Overtight sutures may produce marginal necrosis in the wound at an earlier stage.

427

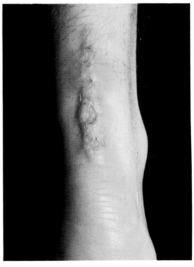

427 Late complication of Achilles tendon surgery. Hypertrophic scar-tissue formation with cracking. It may be treated by injection of steroid directly into the scar or alternatively by wearing an elastic (e.g. 'Jobst') support.

Complications of steroid therapy

Treatment of tendon lesions by steroid injection is contraindicated in view of the strong risk of subsequent tendon rupture. This is particularly exemplified in the Achilles tendon. Even the treatment of peritendonitis by injection may leave chronic deposits in the tissue.

428

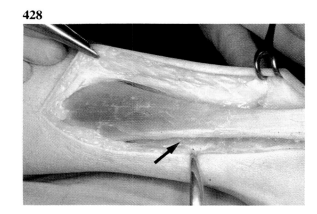

428 Chalky deposits in the paratenon associated with the injection of depot steroid preparations: the tendon itself is intact. Pallor caused by application of tourniquet.

429

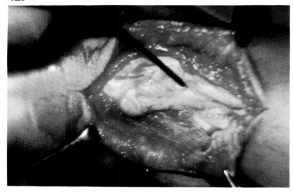

429 Partial rupture of the Achilles tendon due to injection of steroid directly into tendon.

430

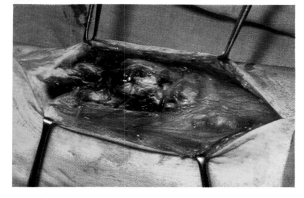

430 Complete rupture of Achilles tendon due to injection of steroid directly into tendon.

16   Ankle injuries

Congenital abnormalities

Congenital abnormalities cause problems by their mechanical interference with the full range of joint movement.

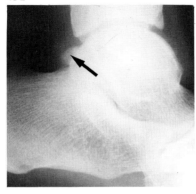

431 Prominent talar spur. Radiographic appearance (see **434**).

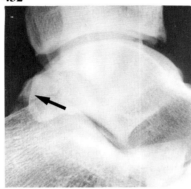

432 Os trigonum – a radiograph. (Note also small impingement exostosis on anterior margin of tibia.) This was causing pain and impaired performance in an international decathlete.

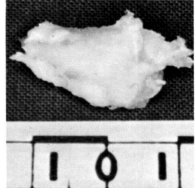

433 Specimen (**432**) after operative removal. The joint between the os trigonum and the talus may show evidence of chondromalacia.

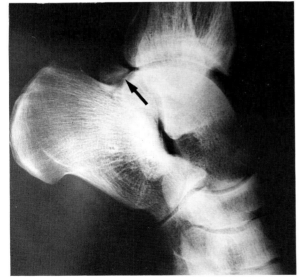

434   Mechanics of interference. The os trigonum (or posterior talar spur) becomes the nut in the nutcracker of the tibia and calcaneum in forced flexion.

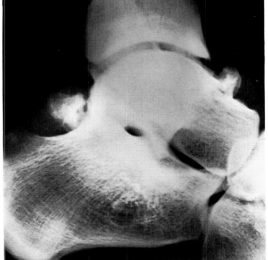

435   Impingement exostosis on calcaneum (note also similar exostosis on talus).

Ankle injury

Ankle injury is common in sport, being often associated with unsuitable footwear. It is particularly seen in football and skiing and ranges in severity from fracture dislocation to simple ligament sprain.

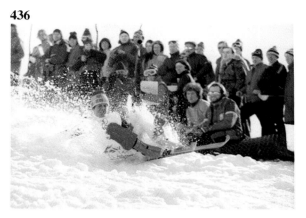

436

436 Skiing accidents are a potent cause of major ankle injuries, particularly if the boots rather than the bindings give way.

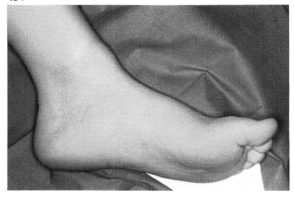

437

437 Fracture dislocation of the ankle joint. Clinical appearance.

Sprains

The 'typical' sprain of the ankle involves the lateral collateral ligament as a result of an inversion injury. Other sprains are relatively unusual.

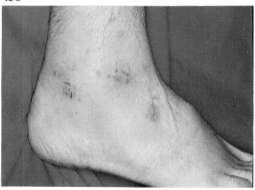

438

438 Simple sprain of the lateral ligament. Clinical appearance.

Sprain of the lateral ligament of the ankle is the most common injury.

Types of sprain

439 'Internal' associated with haemarthrosis. No gross external swelling. **'External'** associated with marked swelling and external bruising.

Some ankle sprains appear very severe when there is gross swelling and ecchymosis, although these are often cases in which the least significant damage is done. The possibility of associated bone injury must always be remembered. Demonstration of clinical instability may require examination under a general anaesthetic with stress x-rays or screening.

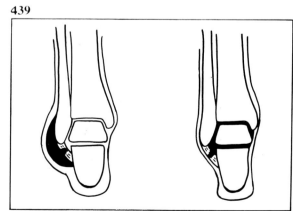

439

'External' sprain
Large bruise
No haemarthrosis
Lateral swelling

'Internal' sprain
Minimal bruise
Haemarthrosis
Posterior swelling

440

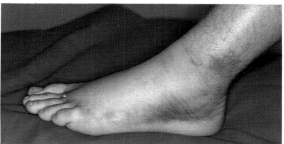

440 An 'external' type of lateral collateral ligament sprain showing dramatic appearance.

441

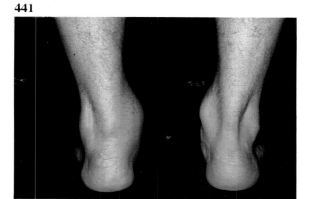

441 Internal type of ankle sprain. Clinical appearance. Swelling is only really noticeable behind the ankle joint due to bulging of the posterior capsule under the pressure of the haemarthrosis which produces swelling on both sides of the Achilles tendon.

442 a

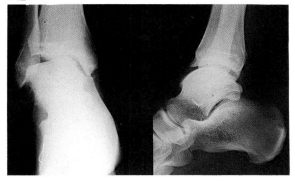

442 a and b In severe cases damage to supporting ligaments will cause the ligament to give way and the joint to become unstable. Stress radiographs showing (a) talar tilt in tear of the lateral collateral ligament and (b) subluxation of the talus (forward tilt) in posterior capsular tear – a forced dorsiflexion injury in a young gymnast.

Note: the ankle is commonly a site of 'stable instability'.

442 b

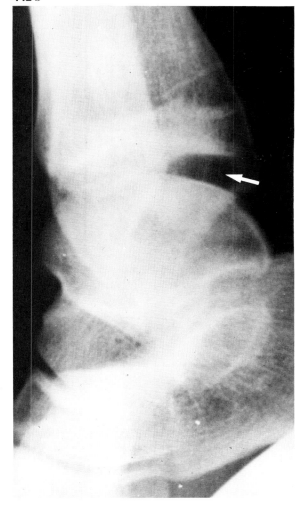

Degenerative joint disease

Clinically the joint may appear normal or there may be visible and palpable thickening. Crepitus is sometimes marked and there may be obvious limitation of movement.

Radiology

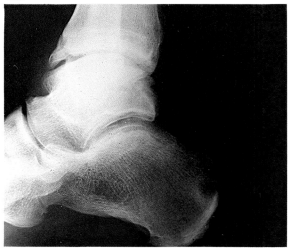

443 Osteoarthrosis. Typical appearance of degenerative joint disease of the ankle joint with narrowing of the joint space and marginal osteophyte formation.

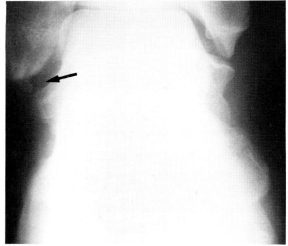

444 'Joint mice'. Minute loose body in ankle joint in a young middle-distance runner.

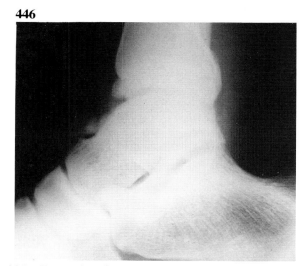

445 Footballer's ankle. Impingement exostoses and marginal osteophyte formation.

Note: the normal joint gap: this is *not* degenerative joint disease and the articular cartilage is not thinned. There is also an os trigonum present which in this case may be an old fractured talar spur.

446 Example of solitary impingement exostosis on the neck of the talus with osteophytes also showing on the anterior aspect of the lower tibia.

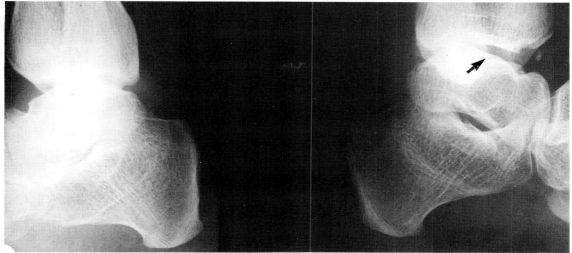

447 Osteochondritis dissecans showing distortion of the talus.

448

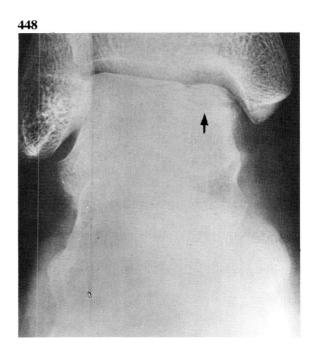

448 Anteroposterior view showing fragment separate from talus.

Osteochondritis dissecans is an uncommon cause of loose-body formation in the ankle joint – the most common cause is post-traumatic osteo-arthrosis. Loose bodies in the ankle joint may cause considerable disability by jamming in the mortice: even very small loose bodies can cause severe symptoms. Treatment is surgical removal.

Heel

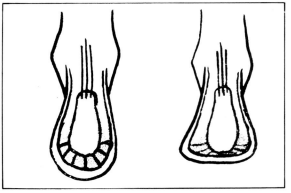

449

449 Heel-bruising mechanism. Note a stress fracture of the calcaneum is occasionally demonstrable.

451 Plantar fasciitis. Diagram to show clinical features and differential diagnosis.

Both calcaneal spur and plantar fasciitis respond to the provision of a high-arch valgus insole with substantial heel padding, ultrasonics, or anti-inflammatory medication topical or systemic. Chronic cases require surgery.

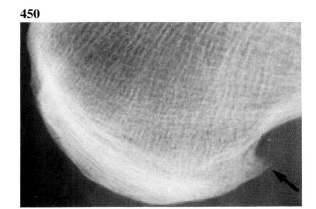

450

450 Calcaneal spur. Radiological appearance.

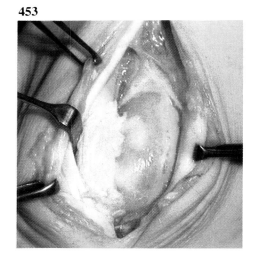

451

Spring ligament sprain   Plantar fasciitis

Tendon lesions

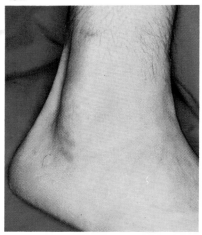

452

452 Snapping or subluxing peroneal tendons. Clinical appearance.

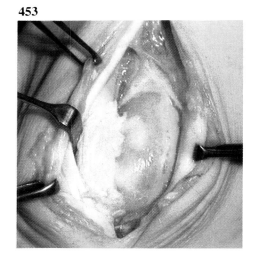

453

453 Subluxing peroneal tendon. Appearance at operation showing degenerated tendon and grossly widened tendon sheath.

454

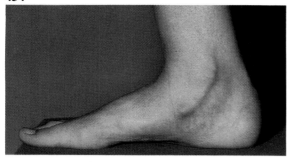

454 Posterior tibial tendovaginitis showing well marked tendon with thickened sheath.

455 Calcification in tendon. Calcification shown in the tendon of peroneus brevis just proximal to insertion.

455

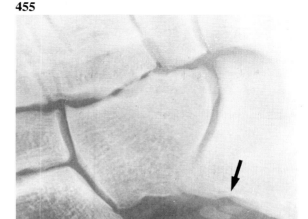

456

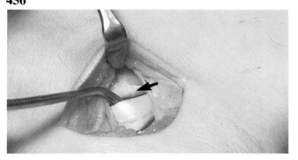

456 Tendovaginitis of extensor hallucis longus. At operation showing thickened tendon sheath.

457

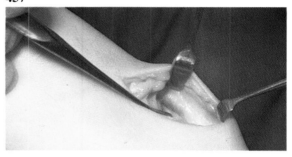

457 Extensor retinaculum entrapment syndrome. Operation for decompression showing muscle fibres inserting into the tendon *distal* to the retinaculum.

458

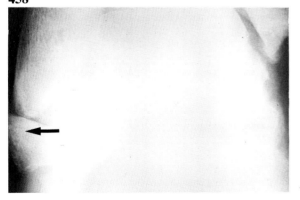

458 Peroneus brevis calcification. Not an accessory ossicle, but calcification in the tendon of peroneus brevis.

459

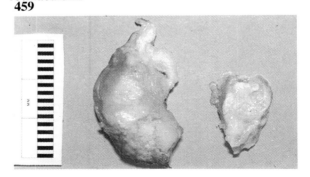

459 Operation specimen from **458**.

Overuse injuries of the stirrup muscle tendons and their sheaths are common about the ankle and often associated with functional deformity of the foot, particularly collapse of the transverse arch.

Treatment, whether conservative or surgical, will often involve the provision of an orthosis to hold the foot in a neutral position and support the collapsing ray while the muscle regains its tone.

17 Foot injuries

Abnormalities

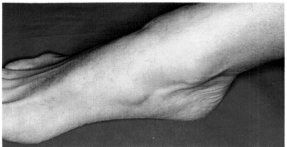

460   Radiograph of foot showing calcaneonavicular bar. A cause of spastic flat foot.

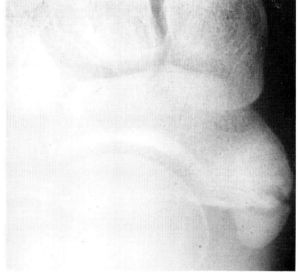

461   Clinical appearance of navicular ossicle showing prominence over the navicular on medial side of foot. This causes pain due to arthrosis in articulation with the main bone.

462   Radiograph showing os naviculare. An accessory ossicle on the navicular.

Tarsal abnormalities are occasionally met and may be a cause of so-called 'spastic flat foot'. As a rule simple supportive measures are all that is needed but where the abnormality is biomechanically significant surgical intervention may be required or the patient may have to give up vigorous sporting activity.

Tarsal fractures/dislocations

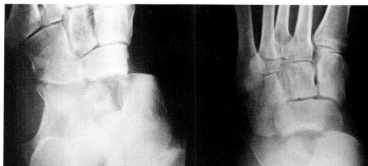

463   Radiograph showing mid-tarsal dislocation in a patient after an accident motor-cycle scrambling.

Tarsal injuries should be treated by rest and support in the early stages, and, after the pain has subsided, by appropriate mobilisation including attention to intrinsic muscle build-up.

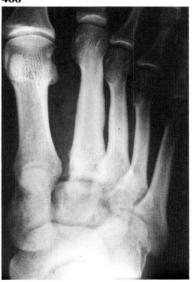

464 Stress fracture of navicular in a young track athlete. A cause for foot pain often misdiagnosed as often not recognised.

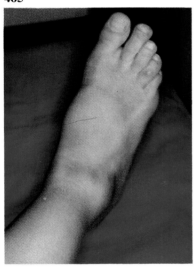

466 Radiological appearance of 465.

465 Gymnast's foot after subluxation of medial ray in a bad landing from a vault. Clinical appearance.

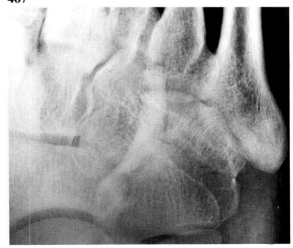

467 Fracture of cuboid. An unusual football injury.

Flatfoot

Postural abnormalities of the foot should not be treated for their own sake, but only if they are associated with significant symptom production (whether in the foot or higher in the leg).

468

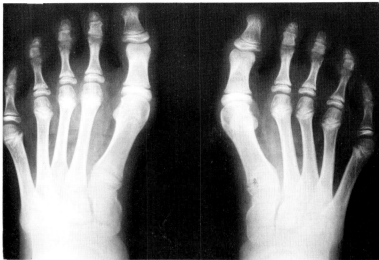

468   Radiograph of broad foot showing metatarsus primus varus. When this condition is well marked a corrective osteotomy may be necessary. Patients with as broad a foot as this need specially fitting shoes.

469

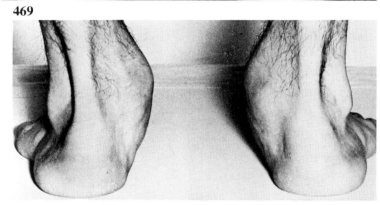

469   Clinical photograph of valgus ankles associated with flatfoot. Note inward lean of the posterior calcaneum.

470

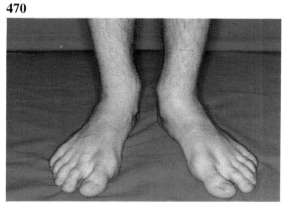

470   Flatfoot in a patient with torsion of the tibia.
Note: The flat appearance of the foot is of no clinical significance if function is good and the subject symptom-free.

471

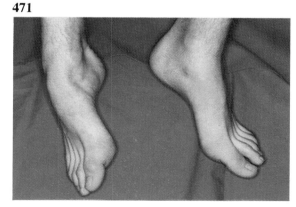

471   Spastic foot. Hardly flat! A spastic foot held in inversion in a young athlete. A psychosomatic disturbance.

Osteochondritis

Osteochondritis is a relatively common cause of localised pain in the foot in sportsmen.

472

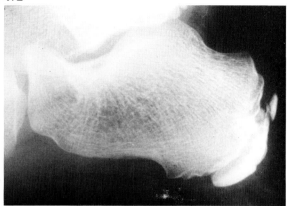

472 Sever's disease. Osteochondritis of the calcaneal apophysis.

Note: Radiological appearances are very variable – this is really a *clinical* diagnosis. It appears to be an overuse traction lesion in adolescents.

473

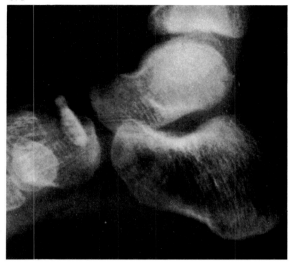

473 Kohler's disease. Osteochondritis of the tarsal navicular leading to distortion of the bone.

474 a

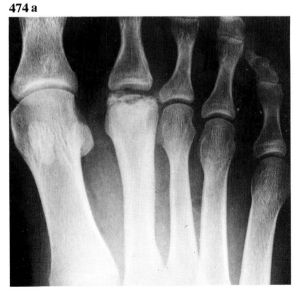

474 b

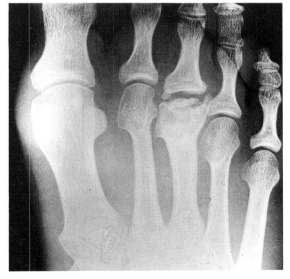

474 a and b Freiburg's disease of the metatarsal heads. Symptoms are due to arthrosis associated with incongruity of distorted joint surfaces.

Osteochondritis in the bones of the foot should be treated by rest. In Kohler's disease in particular distortion and subsequent osteoarthrosis frequently follows over-energetic mobilisation while the disease is active.

Fractures of metatarsals, etc.

Metatarsal injuries are quite common in sport and are often of the overuse type. Chronic forefoot strain or metatarsalgia with no evidence of bone injury is often the result of exercise in unsuitable footwear on terrain to which the sportsman is not accustomed. Clinical features are pain but there are no obvious physical signs.

475

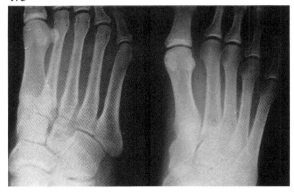

475 In early cases of stress fracture radiological change may be minimal (see **478**). This patient, a gymnast, presented with a history of three weeks pain.

476

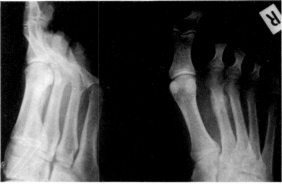

476   Stress fracture of 2nd metatarsal.

477

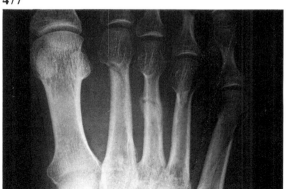

477   Stress fracture of 3rd metatarsal.

478

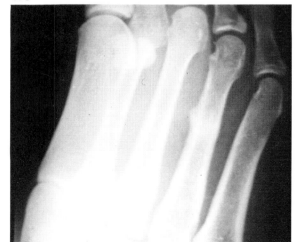

478   Stress fracture of the 4th metatarsal. This radiograph was taken three weeks after that in **475**.

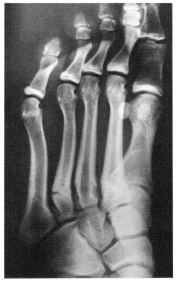

479 Fracture at proximal end of the 4th metatarsal. Cause uncertain. Compare with Jones' fracture (**481**).

480

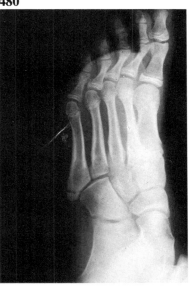

480 Fracture 5th metatarsal styloid due to avulsion stress.

481

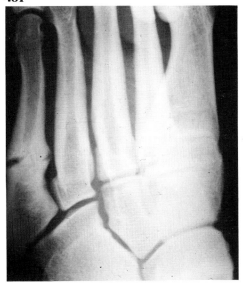

481 Jones' fracture 5th metatarsal styloid. Another stress injury.

482

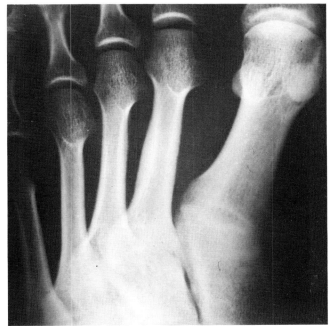

482 Cortical hypertrophy as an alternative stress response in second metatarsal.

Metatarsalgia: other causes

Morton's metatarsalgia is an important cause of pain due to a neuroma developing on the interdigital nerve associated with rubbing between the metatarsal heads.

Treatment of metatarsalgia is essentially the treatment of cause. In functional metatarsalgia associated with overuse, contrast baths, supporting insoles (orthoses) and intrinsic muscle build-up is the treatment of choice.

483

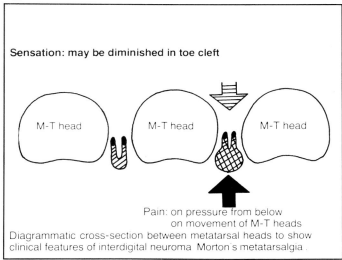

Sensation: may be diminished in toe cleft

M-T head   M-T head   M-T head

Pain: on pressure from below
on movement of M-T heads
Diagrammatic cross-section between metatarsal heads to show clinical features of interdigital neuroma (Morton's metatarsalgia).

483   Interdigital neuroma. Clinical features.

484a

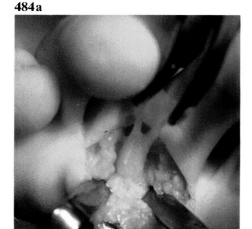

484b

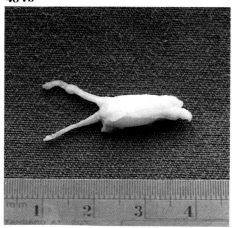

485

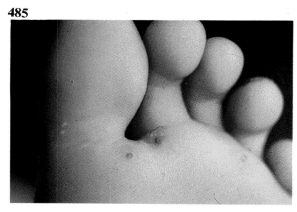

485   Verruca vulgaris. A condition which is often overlooked, but a very important cause of forefoot pain. It is due to a virus infection and may be highly contagious.

484   Interdigital neuroma. a) at operation and **b)** an operative specimen. Note: fusiform swelling on nerve and peripheral branches to contiguous toes.

Blisters

Blisters are often caused by ill-fitted shoes.

486

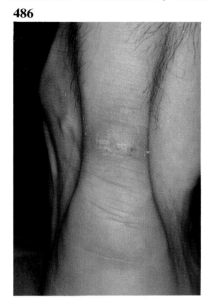

486   Blister. Too stiff a heel counter and tab rub on the tendo Achilles.

488   Blister. A stud or spike pushing through from below rubs under the forefoot.

Blisters are readily treated by removing the dead skin and applying adhesive plaster directly over the raw area. It sounds drastic but is effective and remarkably comfortable for the patient.

487

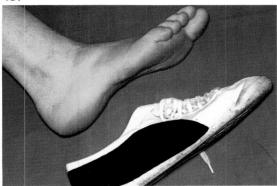

487   Blister. A broad foot needs a wide-fitting shoe. Sports footwear should be manufactured in a variety of fittings.

488

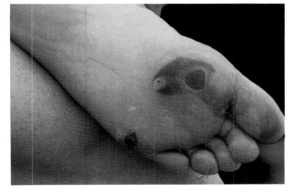

Some oddities

489

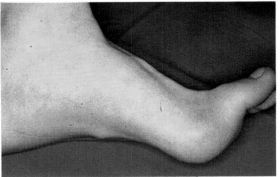

489   Inclusion dermoid in the sole of the foot.

490

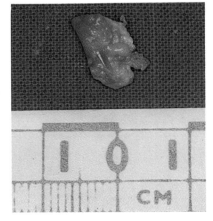

490   Fragment of artificial turf removed with inclusion dermoid from the foot.

491

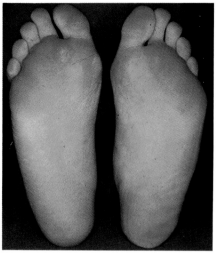

491   Deep vein thrombosis in the plantar veins of the foot (due to unaccustomed exercise on a very hard floor surface).

492

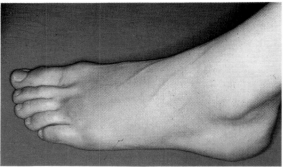

492   Extensor tenosynovitis on dorsum of foot (often due to bad lacing of shoes). To avoid unsatisfactory distribution of pressure, shoes with a long throat (i.e. with more than 3 lace holes) should be laced with 2 laces, the proximal laces being tied tightly, the distal laces being tied loosely.

493

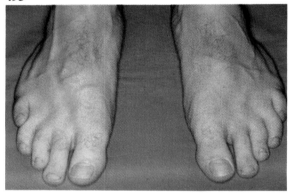

493   Congenital abnormality. Note alignment of 4th and little toes! This shape of foot is of academic rather than clinical significance but may produce problems in shoe fitting.

Toe injuries

494

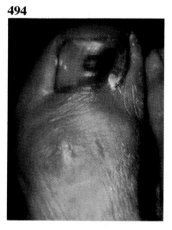

494   Subungual haematoma due to direct violence. A similar condition, resulting from ill-fitting shoes, is often seen affecting the toe-nails of the 1st and 2nd toes in long-distance runners.

495

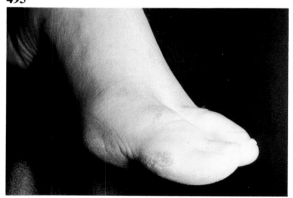

495   Callosity on the medial aspect of the toe and under the 1st metatarsophalangeal joint. Result of ill-fitting shoes in a long-distance runner.

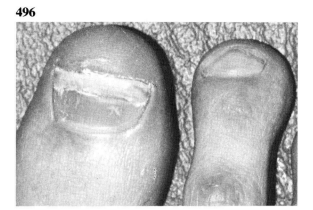

496 Nail-bed damage to great toenail due to ill-fitting shoes.

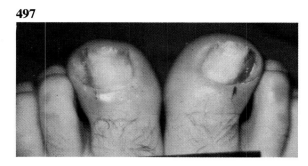

497 Ingrowing toenails. A common clinical problem in sportsmen.

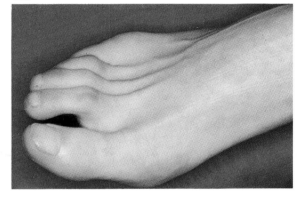

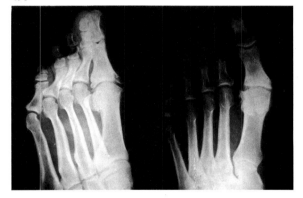

498 and 499 Hallux rigidus in middle-distance runner. Clinical and radiological appearances. This condition may be extremely difficult to treat and the victim often has to abandon his athletic career prematurely.

Morton's foot

In many subjects the first metatarsal is shorter than the second (Morton's foot). It is argued that this particular arrangement with a long second toe makes the subject more prone to stress fractures of the metatarsals and to sesamoiditis, but this has not been confirmed in controlled studies. However, Morton's foot does make the management of hallux rigidus more difficult. The latter can be treated conservatively by manipulation under a general anaesthetic and/or intra-articular steroid injections. In some cases a metatarsal bar may be helpful but this will often interfere with foot function in sporting activity. Surgical treatment is unfortunately often ineffective in allowing return to sport.

500

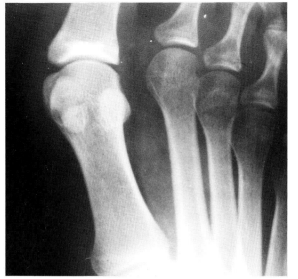

500 Sesamoiditis. Radiograph showing disruption of the medial sesamoid under the first metatarsal head. Anteroposterior radiograph.

501

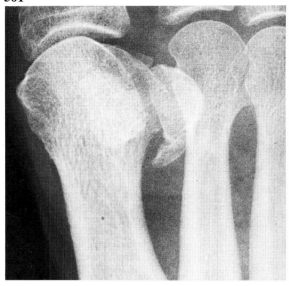

501 Sesamoiditis. Old appearances with marginal osteophyte formation. Oblique radiograph. Sesamoiditis is often due to inadequate padding or protection in the sole of the shoe or boot.

502

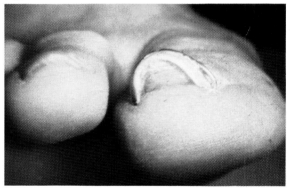

502 Subungual exostosis. Clinical appearance.

503

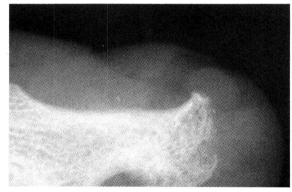

503 Subungual exostosis. Radiographic appearance.
The cause is uncertain; the treatment surgical, radical and usually very effective.

504

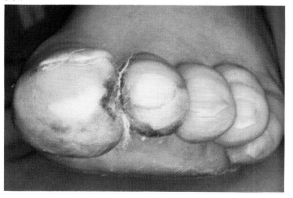

504 Cold injury. Frostbite due to inadequate ski boots. Another, and rather unusual, example of the consequences of unsatisfactory footwear.

Further reading

The following English language publications may be useful:

Journals

American Journal of Sports Medicine, 105 Physicians Building, Columbus, GA 31901, USA

British Journal of Sports Medicine, 39 Linkfield Road, Mountsorrel, Nr Loughborough, Leics

Journal of Sports Medicine and Physical Fitness, Corso Bramante 83–85, 10126 Torino, Italy

Medicine and Science in Sports, 1440 Monroe Street, Madison, Wisconsin 53706, USA

Medisport, Howmedica Publications, 1 Packhorse Road, Gerrards Cross, Bucks

Physician and Sportsmedicine, 4530 West 77th Street, Minneapolis 55435, USA

Books

Gibbs, R., *Sports Injuries*, MacMillan Company of Australia Pty Ltd

Muckle, D. S., *Injuries in Sport*, John Wright & Sons, Bristol

O'Donoghue, D. H., *Treatment of Injuries to Athletes* (3rd Ed), W. B. Saunders Company, Philadelphia

Problems of Sports Medicine and Sports Training and Coaching, and *Basic Book of Sports Medicine*, Olympic Solidarity, available through National Olympic Committees

Quigley, T. B. (Editor), *Year Book of Sports Medicine*, New York Medical Publishers Inc., Chicago and London

Allman, F. L., and Ryan, A. J., *Sports Medicine*, Academic Press, London and New York

Williams, J. G. P., and Sperryn, P. N., *Sports Medicine* (2nd Ed), Edward Arnold, London

Index